DEAFNESS, COMMUNITY AND CULTURE IN BRITAIN

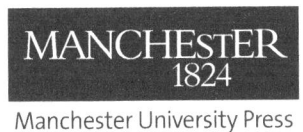

MANCHESTER
1824

Manchester University Press

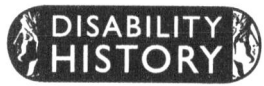

Dr Julie Anderson, Professor Walton Schalick, III

This new series published by Manchester University Press responds to the growing interest in disability as a discipline worthy of historical research. The series has a broad international historical remit, encompassing issues that include class, race, gender, age, war, medical treatment, professionalization, environments, work, institutions and cultural and social aspects of disablement including representations of disabled people in literature, film, art and the media.

DEAFNESS, COMMUNITY AND CULTURE IN BRITAIN

LEISURE AND COHESION, 1945–1995

Martin Atherton

Manchester University Press

Published by Manchester University Press
Altrincham Street, Manchester M1 7JA, UK
www.manchesteruniversitypress.co.uk

British Library Cataloguing-in-Publication Data is available

Library of Congress Cataloging-in-Publication Data is available

ISBN 978 0 7190 9978 6   paperback

First published by Manchester University Press in hardback 2012

This edition first published 2016

Printed by Lightning Source

With grateful thanks to the staff of
English Martyrs Primary School, Preston,
1963–1967

Contents

List of tables

List of figures

Acknowledgements

In producing this book and the research it is based upon, I received invaluable help and assistance from a number of people. Richard Holt, Mike Cronin and Jeff Hill were particularly important supporters during their time with the International Centre for Sports History and Culture at De Montfort University, Leicester, as were my former colleagues Dave Russell and John Walton at the University of Central Lancashire. Thanks are also due to Martin Polley of the University of Southampton and John Hay at the University of Wolverhampton. Special mention must go to Julie Anderson of the University of Kent for her unwavering friendship and support and to my editor at Manchester University Press, Emma Brennan. Finally, but most importantly of all, I would like to offer my immense gratitude to all those contributors, most of whom will remain forever anonymous, who reported their deaf clubs' activities in the pages of *British Deaf News*. In doing so, they provided an historical record of the deaf community that is both unique and invaluable. I hope that I have used their insights into deaf life in a way they would find interesting.

List of abbreviations

AADD	The Association in Aid of the Deaf and Dumb
ASL	American Sign Language
BDA	British Deaf Association
BDASA	British Deaf Amateur Sports Association
BDN	*British Deaf News*
BDSC	British Deaf Sports Council
BDT	*British Deaf Times*
BSL	British Sign Language
BWSF	British Workers' Sport Federation
CDA	Catholic Deaf Association
CHA	The Co-operative Holidays Association
CISS	Comite Internationale des Sports des Sourds
CIU	Club and Institute Union
DHA	Disability History Association
DWEB	Deaf Welfare Examination Board
DWO	Deaf Welfare Officer
EDGA	English Deaf Golf Association
FLCD	Federation of London Deaf Clubs
IPC	International Paralympic Committee
NWDSA	North West Deaf Sports Association
NWDSC	North West Deaf Sports Council
RAD	Royal Association in Aid of Deaf People
RNID	Royal National Institute for Deaf People

1

INTRODUCTION

When, as a mature student, I began reading for a degree in Deaf Studies and History in the 1990s, my tutors regularly told me that deaf clubs were vital to the existence and continuation of the British deaf community. This was confirmed by my reading of academic literature, which consistently emphasised that the deaf club has long been the place in which deaf people gathered together and where deaf culture was celebrated and enjoyed.[1] However, neither my tutors nor the books and articles I read could answer what were for me key questions in helping me understand what forms this celebration of 'deaf culture' took: where were these clubs located? How many of them were there? Who attended them and who ran them? Most importantly of all, what did deaf people do there? The only clues were vague ones: 'deaf people like to gather together in the clubs, tell stories, pass on their shared history and swap jokes about and against the hearing world'. That was virtually all the detail I could find and the more I searched the more obvious it became that there is very little known outside the community about what actually went on in the deaf clubs. I was constantly asking myself, 'If deaf culture is so important and deaf clubs are a central venue for its expression, then what precisely did this "deaf culture" consist of? What did the deaf clubs provide for their members that made them so important?' This book sets out to address this lack of knowledge by providing the first extensive examination of the nature and detail of deaf communal life in Britain. I do not claim that this study will provide a full and definitive explanation of everything that might be represented by the terms 'deaf community' and 'deaf culture'; there are at least as many definitions of these as there are people with opinions on these matters. What it does do is offer some previously hidden insights into what life was like for deaf people in post-war Britain, in terms of their leisure choices and opportunities for spending their free time. This results in a more detailed understanding of how deaf people interacted with each other and the surrounding hearing world, the social and cultural behaviour of British deaf people in leisure settings, and how this interaction influenced their perceptions of their deafness as a factor in their individual and collective identities.

Focusing on the period since the end of the Second World War, this study uncovers the reality of communal life for deaf club members in the UK, and draws on a detailed case study of north-west England to illustrate broader trends and patterns in deaf socialisation and to locate these activities within theoretical constructions of leisure practices and motivations. Focusing on one region of Britain provides an opportunity to more closely examine the realities of deaf leisure and its meanings and importance in the lives of British deaf people. Although there were some minor regional differences in the way deaf people shared their leisure lives, there was a large degree of consistency and homogeneity in the types of activities deaf club members chose to take part in and a detailed national survey of deaf leisure would prove both unwieldy and unnecessary. I chose to focus on the north-west for a variety of reasons, not least because that is where I live and work, but there are also other considerations than mere geographical convenience. With its wide variety of urban and rural settings, north-west England provides examples of the different types of social settings deaf people found themselves in across Britain. From the isolated towns of Cumbria and north Lancashire to the close networks of factory towns of east and central Lancashire, through the coalfields in the south-west of the region to the large cities of Manchester and Liverpool and their satellite towns, north-west England serves as a microcosm of all aspects of the wider deaf experience in post-war Britain. In addition, there are a large number of deaf clubs within the region (twenty-eight in all), again representing the variety of urban locations found nationally. By focusing on the north-west as a representative sample of the lived deaf experience, a much more detailed and revealing insight into deaf leisure practices can be achieved. Whilst some of the statistics and rates of participation might have varied between different parts of the country, the underlying patterns, motivations and rewards of shared leisure lives were the same.

The question of 'Who are these people we call deaf?' needs to be answered before any assessment of their social lives can be made and the extensive literature on deafness is analysed in order to attempt to address this question. In the early years of the twenty-first century, deafness and deaf people are more obvious and noticeable in many aspects of British life than ever before. Many of the rights of deaf people, particularly sign language users, are enshrined and protected in law and focused services are available in a variety of settings. Yet despite all this apparent public awareness, deafness is still seen as a disability and deaf people continue to suffer from the negative perceptions that arise as a consequence. Deaf people are not unusual in being seen as being disabled; many other groups and individuals within society are identified on the basis of particular physical or mental health characteristics. This view is based on long established medical models of disability, which have concentrated on notions of 'loss' or 'abnormality', as will be explained in later chapters. Such people have to some extent been placed on the fringes of mainstream society, if not completely removed from common perceptions of community and society. The idea that people sharing similar conditions or disabilities might constitute a community is a recent development and such notions are not fully or generally understood.[2] As a result of these perceptions, disabled people found a rare if somewhat perverse example of equality in their treatment as suitable subjects for historical research and discourse. They have been largely absent from social or cultural history until comparatively recently and when they did appear disabled people were almost invariably portrayed from a perspective that concentrates on medical aspects and conceptions of disability. However, this imbalance has been redressed in recent years, with an increasing caucus of research that approaches perceptions of disability from a social and cultural perspective.[3] The emergence of organisations such as the Disability History Association in the US and the Disability History Group in the UK and Europe demonstrates the development of these branches of historical research and has helped to stimulate interest in rediscovering the social history of such groups, rather than merely their medical conditions and impairments.

One such group that has developed a broader collective identity based on a more positive perception of deafness is that most commonly known as 'the deaf community'. The existence of a distinct and identifiable deaf community has been acknowledged for a number of years and these debates have begun to become more widely accepted (if not necessarily understood) within the public consciousness.[4] Various models by which membership of the deaf community may be conferred or attained were devised and ways in which deaf people expressed their shared social and cultural identity were identified as a result of these discussions.[5] This community is not comprised of people who view themselves as disabled by their inability to hear; instead the deaf community sees itself as having a distinct social, cultural and linguistic foundation that results from community members being deaf. In doing so, those people who constitute the deaf community accept and celebrate their deafness as a positive element of their lives. It is these people and this community that are the focus of this book. The cultural aspects of the deaf community are not seen by its members to be in any way 'abnormal'; they are merely responses to the specific requirements for communication and socialisation that result from shared deafness. As a consequence, many authors have sought ways to define the structure and culture of the deaf community in terms that reject the concept of deafness as a disability.[6] For those readers new to the academic field of Deaf Studies, these models and the debates they have generated are unpacked in chapter two. These debates will demonstrate that even defining 'deafness' from a social perspective is fraught with difficulties. Determining who should then be regarded as belonging within the deaf community and to what extent continues to exercise academics, theorists and deaf activists and despite the best efforts of many commentators, no definitive answers have emerged. Nor does it seem possible that any definition that would reflect and encompass the full range of views and opinions is ever achievable. Nevertheless these arguments and models are explored to give a flavour of the complexity of deaf identity on both personal and communal levels.

As a result of the raised awareness of deaf community as both a concept and a reality (both internally and amongst the general population), interest in uncovering the hidden history of deafness and deaf people from a social and cultural perspective has grown since the last quarter of the twentieth century and is now the focus of much research.[7] Even so, much of what passes for deaf history remains more concerned with recounting the histories of important places, organisations or individuals, rather than any detailed reconstruction of the lives of the people who made up the deaf community. These discussions and affirmations on the cultural aspects of deafness have been made without the support of any quantifiable evidence of the deaf community's main form of cultural expression – the shared leisure activities of its members. Although the deaf community and deaf culture have been defined several times using various criteria, these definitions have not included any quantitative data on the social life of the deaf community. Whilst the extensive discourses on deaf community membership have concentrated on identifying and promoting the distinct elements of deaf life, especially sign language use, and emphasising the importance of the deaf club within the community, this has been done without anything more than a scant acknowledgement of what communal deaf life involved. The lack of empirical evidence to support the definitions of the deaf community suggests that there has been an implicit acceptance of the ways in which the deaf community has spent its communal leisure time and so expressed its shared culture. However, the leisure activities which fall within this area of 'common knowledge' have never been explicitly stated in more than general terms. Nor has a wider view been considered which encompasses those elements of deaf life that do not differ significantly from those of hearing people. This lack of quantitative evidence means there is no data against which to test the validity of these qualitative models as expressions of the realities of deaf life.

One of the main ways in which deaf people spent their leisure time was by becoming members of their local deaf clubs alongside others with similar experiences, interests and outlooks. The history and importance of the deaf clubs will be described, to illustrate the way in which these clubs collectively and individually served as social and cultural hubs for the deaf community. Deaf clubs developed as the social arms of the voluntary welfare organisations for deaf people that emerged from the mid-nineteenth century onwards. An important but previously unconsidered factor in this development of both welfare and social bodies for deaf people was the impact of the Poor Law Amendment Act of 1834 on deaf people. Placed in an invidious position by the concepts of 'deserving poor' and 'undeserving poor' introduced by the Act, many deaf people found themselves subjected to the iniquities of the new, stricter workhouse regimes. The ways in which Victorian philanthropists sought to save deaf people from this fate and the consequences of their actions on the formation and maintenance of a deaf community in Britain are explored here.

Once the provenance of deaf clubs, and by extension the British deaf community, has been established, the shared social lives of deaf club members can be identified and assessed. Precisely what these social and sporting activities were and how they helped in the development and maintenance of a community of deaf people, has never been investigated in such detail before. Revealing the precise nature of these activities provides fresh insights into not only the leisure choices of deaf people but also their relationships with each other and with those amongst whom they lived – the hearing world.

Hill and Williams advocated taking both 'empiricist' and 'reflectionist' approaches as a methodology for dealing with the social history of leisure, and this strategy has been employed in order to identify both quantitative and qualitative issues of deaf leisure.[8] The resulting data is used throughout this book to illustrate both the social choices made by deaf people and the motivations behind these choices. The case study considers the reported activities of the members of twenty-eight deaf clubs over a period of fifty years, which provided a combination of latitudinal and longitudinal data. Not everything that might be considered deaf leisure has been identified; nor is it claimed that all the activities organised by deaf clubs were reported in *British Deaf News*. The source materials simply cannot and do not provide such a minutely detailed record. However, the large body of evidence gathered has allowed specific patterns and trends in deaf leisure to be identified and a number of qualitative factors relating to issues of motivation, preference and choice have emerged. As the data was drawn from deaf newspapers and specifically reports submitted by deaf club members themselves, the argument is put forward that the data accurately portrays the views and preferences of those people considered by this investigation. These data thus reflect internal perceptions of deaf leisure choices, as well as allowing externally generated conclusions on these factors of deaf life to be reached. As will be demonstrated in chapter five, newspapers published specifically for a deaf readership have played an important role in maintaining contact across the deaf community. In many ways, they provided the only medium for the large scale dissemination of news, opinions and information between deaf people until the introduction of technology that was not reliant on sound and voice as a means of communication. Prior to the widespread availability of textphones, mobile phones, email and the internet, deaf people were largely reliant on face to face contact for local news and deaf newspapers for a larger geographical perspective on deaf issues that rarely – if ever – featured in the mainstream media. It was not until the British Broadcasting Corporation launched *See Hear* in 1981 that deaf people had their own dedicated television magazine programme, but even this only ran for thirty minutes a week for part of the year. Although *See Hear* served an important cultural role, not least in making deaf people more visible on national television, the limitations of time and format meant it could do little more than supplement deaf newspapers as a medium for disseminating information to and about deaf people. The fact that it was the readership who were contributing large sections of these papers only adds to their value as a unique and invaluable historical resource.

In some respects, newspapers for deaf readers have served a similar purpose to local newspapers and have closely reflected the perspectives of the community. Whilst certain sections of these newspapers sought to inform and more latterly influence opinions amongst their readers, the pages devoted to reports of deaf club news remained very much concerned with reflecting the social lives of deaf club members and disseminating this information nationally. This information thus provides unique and highly personal insights into a range of cultural aspects of deaf communal leisure. This makes these publications an important means of gaining insights into all aspects of the community across a considerable period of time. Many of the issues discussed in this book can be applied to other community groups, with the deafness of the participants being largely inconsequential when applying theoretical concepts of leisure activity to the data. Several of the principles used in this analysis could be equally applied to groups founded on the basis of shared national or ethnic heritage, gender or religious beliefs, or geographical location to name just a few. Knowing how deaf people chose to fill their leisure time may have intrinsic interest and value in its own right, but as Richard Holt has argued, it is necessary to consider specific groups and communities within a conceptual framework.[9] The case study of north-west England therefore commences with a brief history of leisure and sport in the region from 1945 onwards, through which broader influences on the leisure choices and practices of deaf people can be identified and their cultural influences examined. This is underpinned by a discussion of the role of leisure generally and sport in particular in the development of structured and identifiable communities. In this way, concepts relating to deaf leisure are illustrated within a wider contextualisation of socialisation and community formation across the north west, and the deaf community serves as an example of leisure development and purpose for many other groups in the region. The deaf community provides a rare opportunity to analyse an identifiable social group comprising a significant number of people, spread over an extensive geographical area, and spanning a period of half a century. The amount of data and detail that this breadth of investigation has uncovered makes it unique in its scope, and of value and interest to a wide range of social historians. That the group being considered were deaf people is not particularly significant in this respect; it is their communal social activities that are of primary importance, as this provides a basis to investigate issues of community formation, maintenance and cohesion that can be applied more widely. This study thus contributes to a greater appreciation of the social history of the deaf community on a national basis and to a broader understanding of the leisure history of north-west England in the post-war period.

The methods of defining the deaf community outlined earlier and examined in more detail in the following chapter have been largely unchallenged since the mid 1980s. Therefore the criteria for determining how membership should be assigned and recognised will be tested against the historical record provided by *British Deaf News*, to assess the veracity of these models from a historical point of view. Does the history of deaf leisure support or challenge the theoretical assumptions made about what becoming a member of a deaf community involved, through active membership of a deaf club? The history of deaf leisure provides evidence of the ways in which deaf club members remained fairly constant in terms of their leisure choices, whilst at the same time the very structure of the deaf community was undergoing a period of unprecedented change and upheaval. Communal deaf life has changed irrevocably during the post-war period and the evidence presented in this study suggests ways in which it may continue to evolve in the future (although it must be acknowledged that attempting to project and predict is always a dangerous activity for historians). Various examples found in the historical record raise questions about the very nature of the deaf community, its composition and its culture. Examples such as the activities of Bolton deaf club members, who were making theatre and cinema trips in the 1960s, and the promotion of pop concerts at Liverpool deaf club in the same period challenge theories about precisely who was involved in these events and consequently who should be included when considering membership of the deaf community. One of the findings proposed from analysis of such events is that all those who took part in deaf club events should be considered to be members of the deaf community to some extent and that anything deaf people chose to do together should be considered as elements of deaf culture. Whilst I accept that not everyone may agree with these arguments and that they might seem controversial or even heretical to some, the evidence indicates that deaf culture, when defined as the leisure activities that deaf people freely chose to engage in, has been much more integrated with hearing culture than the existing literature suggests.

Some commentators have given broad examples of the way deaf culture was expressed within the deaf clubs, but there has been no evidence of how else deaf people spent their leisure time.[10] There is certainly no indication that certain aspects of communal deaf leisure (and by extension deaf culture) were the same as those enjoyed by non-deaf people, or that deaf people may have taken part in certain activities for reasons other than being deaf. By investigating more closely which leisure activities deaf people chose to take part in together, a greater insight into the way deaf people followed wider patterns of social and cultural behaviour becomes evident. This allows a fresh perspective on the distinctiveness and conformity of deaf leisure to be obtained; for example, the influence of 'Beatlemania' and the 'Merseybeat' in the 1960s can be clearly seen in the events organised for young deaf Liverpudlians at that time and this challenges some interpretations of what should – and should not – be considered as 'deaf culture'. Subtle changes in the way deaf club members gradually became the providers – rather than the sole recipients – of charitable donations derived from social events can also be seen in the context of an increasing political awareness amongst deaf people.

As part of this process, the way in which deaf people replicated the leisure and sporting activities of other communities within society will be demonstrated. In turn, this conformity of leisure has important implications when the issue of whether deafness should be considered as a disability is raised at the conclusion of this book. In many respects, deaf people have shown themselves to be no different to anyone else in the ways in which they have chosen to fill their spare time, and evidence to support this conclusion will be presented throughout this study. This evidence also illuminates trends in community development that are found across society. For example, Puttnam contends that social networks have altered and fragmented since the Second World War, and the analysis of the deaf community will be shown to support many (but not all) of Puttnam's arguments.[11] The same evidence will also be used to illustrate how ideas of the emergence of nation states put forward by Benedict

Anderson can be seen in the political development of the deaf community.[12] The deaf community will thus be shown to have followed similar paths to other social or cultural groups in certain aspects of its internal structures and patterns of growth.

The concept of topophilia is considered, and arguments are put forward to support the contention that membership of a deaf club represented attachment to a group of people as much as to a physical place, drawing on the work of Bale, Tuan and Wise in particular.[13] 'The deaf club' is generally understood as a particular place where deaf people gathered, rather than being considering as a more nebulous entity that encompasses the wider activities its members took part in as a group. The evidence presented in deaf newspapers and analysed here clearly indicates that deaf club members felt as much attachment to the concept of the deaf club as a group of like-minded people as they did to its physical premises. The deaf club could just as easily be embodied in those members who took part in a particular event or activity, no matter where it took place. So the deaf club as a representation of a much larger 'imagined community' (i.e. the deaf community) could be found on a coach, in a holiday camp or even on board a cruise ship. In many instances, the location was less important in terms of understanding the reality of 'the deaf club' than the people who engaged in a particular activity. In this respect, this study raises questions about deaf people's own understanding of what the deaf club represented in their lives and how this was reflected in their attachments to both people and place.

This book therefore argues that participation in leisure and sport has been a central factor in the development and maintenance of the British deaf community, and that deaf clubs were the main providers and primary means of entry into that communal social life. Whilst leisure and sport activities will be shown to have served specific and vital purposes in establishing social and cultural cohesion within the deaf community, it will be demonstrated that deaf people have not engaged in leisure practices in ways which are significantly different from other sections of the broader population. Certain activities were engaged in more regularly by deaf club members, whilst evidence of other activities (particularly certain sports) is rarely or never found in the deaf newspapers, but it is clear that deaf people did not engage in leisure activities that were markedly different to those of their hearing counterparts. As will be seen throughout this study, it was not merely the types of activities that illustrate the importance of shared social activities to the deaf community. It was the broader social, cultural and psychological benefits of such involvement that made shared leisure and sport such vital components in the establishment and continuation of the deaf community.

The ways in which communal leisure contributed to the formation of group and self-identity are discussed and theories relating to the roles of leisure and sport within communities tested. This process helps to determine if and how leisure in the deaf community may replicate or differ from the roles and purposes such activities serve in other social and community groups. Both the sources used and the data derived from them provide a unique opportunity to gain intimate access to a largely misunderstood and misrepresented community of people and to assess their engagement with each other and with outsiders. This allows questions to be raised not only about what this community did together but equally importantly, why they chose to take part in these activities and what benefits they derived from doing so. As this study shows, many of the activities deaf people enjoyed were the same as those of hearing people. Therefore, deaf people can be used as a case study for investigating the roles of leisure and sport across a variety of social groups. An analysis of deaf people's social lives provides an opportunity to learn more about a minority group who feel themselves to be oppressed and misrepresented by the majority culture (in this instance, non-deaf people). Many members of the deaf community reject external perceptions of deafness and deaf people that are based on medical or pathological models, instead viewing themselves as a social, cultural and linguistic minority. When the history of the leisure lives of deaf club members is uncovered, many of the arguments put forward which claim deaf people are unable to live 'normal' lives because of their perceived 'disability' are challenged. Not only does this study reveal the great extent, variety and popularity of shared leisure activities amongst deaf people, it also demonstrates that, in their leisure lives at least, deaf club members enjoyed precisely the same types of activities as their hearing counterparts, deriving the same social, emotional and psychological benefits in the process and showing themselves to be in no way disadvantaged or disabled. Indeed, the data suggests that deaf club members might have had a more active and rewarding social life than many of their hearing contemporaries, which went beyond merely providing enhanced opportunities for passing free time. This social life also reinforced ideas of shared identity and culture by bringing together an otherwise isolated and dispersed group of people who shared not only similar interests and outlooks but who had also be subjected to a range of negative perceptions and attitudes. Far from being disabled, they were in fact empowered and advantaged through their membership of a deaf club.

The book concludes by considering how the gradual decline of deaf clubs reflects the changing social and political nature of the British deaf community. Since 1995, the end of the period covered by this study, deaf leisure as represented by deaf club activity has come under serious and almost certainly terminal threat. Although no quantifiable data on the demographic structure of deaf club membership since 1995 is available, both anecdotal and direct personal experience indicates that the clubs are increasingly the preserve of older deaf people. The younger elements of the signing population no longer gravitate towards deaf clubs, preferring more mainstream venues and forms of entertainment to the traditional forms of deaf leisure. The sad inevitability is that unless drastic action is taken to attract these younger generations back to the clubs, they will die out with their members. Other than isolated examples, nothing that has happened in the years since 1995 suggests this is a likely outcome, and what this decline means for the future of the deaf community is assessed in the final chapter. Whilst the gradual disappearance of the deaf clubs might be seen as a prime example of Puttnam's theories on the erosion of social networks through the loss of communal leisure, this is not necessarily the case. In many respects, deaf clubs have been the victims of their own success and their time is now past. By bringing deaf people together, they allowed the gradual development of a shared political agenda that has driven the campaign for equality for deaf sign language users. Without a network of venues through which deaf people could become politically active, the empowering process by which younger deaf people no longer feel the need to hide away from the hearing world could not have taken place. It is through the gradual rejection of deafness as a disability that deaf clubs have slowly but surely been replaced as the centres of deaf social life. Deaf communal leisure is not disappearing but it is undergoing a period of radical change. Young deaf people are more confident about celebrating their deafness; they make no apologies for using sign language and at the same time they want to take part in mainstream cultural activities on their own terms. They are more likely to be found in pubs, bars and clubs than their deaf antecedents and much less likely to attend traditional deaf clubs. In doing so, they are reversing the tradition of deaf people wanting their own space away from the hearing world but at the same time they are continuing to make their own choices about how and with whom they spend their free time. There is no doubt that the days of the deaf clubs are numbered but the role they have played in developing and maintaining the deaf community and in helping to improve the lives of deaf people today and in the future cannot be underestimated. How this process has come about is told at least in part in this book.

Notes

1   Harris, Jennifer, *The cultural meaning of deafness* (Aldershot, Avebury, 1995); Kyle and Woll, *Sign language*, p. 11; P. Ladd, 'The modern deaf community' in D. Miles, *BSL, a beginners guide* (London, BBC Books, 1988) pp. 37–38; C. Mason, 'School experiences' in Gregory and Hartley *Constructing deafness* pp. 84–87; C. Padden,

'The deaf community and the culture of deaf people' in S. Wilcox (ed.), *American deaf culture* (Burtonsville: Linstock 1989), pp. 1–16

2   See for example M. Oliver, *The politics of disablement* (London: Macmillan, 1990), pp. 14–17

3   Examples include J. Knight, *Excluding attitudes: disabled people's experience of social exclusion* (London, Leonard Cheshire Foundation, 1999); D.T. Mitchell and S. Snyder, *The body and physical difference: discourses of disability* (Ann Arbor: University of Michigan Press, 1997); J. Swain, S. French and C. Cameron, *Controversial issues in a disabling society* (Buckingham: Open University Press, 2003)

4   For example R. Sutton-Spence and B. Woll, *The linguistics of British Sign Language: an introduction* (Cambridge: Cambridge University Press, 1999); P. Ladd, *Understanding deaf culture: in search of deafhood* (London: Multicultural Matters, 2003)

5   Models of the deaf community include C. Baker-Shenk and D. Cokely, *American Sign Language: a teacher's resource text on curriculum, methods ands evaluation* (Washington DC: Gallaudet University Press, 1980); P. Higgins, *Outsiders in a hearing world* (London: Sage, 1980); L. Lawson, 'The role of sign in the structure of the deaf community' in S. Gregory and G.M. Hartley (eds), *Constructing deafness* (London: Pinter Publishers, 1991) pp. 31–34; C. Padden and T. Humphries, *Deaf in America: voices from a culture* (London: Harvard University Press, 1988)

6   Corker, M., *Deaf and disabled or deafness disabled?* (Buckingham: Open University Press, 1998); V. Finkelstein, 'We are not disabled, you are' in Gregory and Hartley *Constructing deafness* pp. 265–271; P. Ladd, *Understanding deaf culture: in search of deafhood (London: Multicultural Matters, 2003)*

7   Grant, B., *The deaf advance* (Edinburgh: Pentland, 1990); R. Lee (ed.), *Deaf liberation* (London: National Union of the Deaf, 1992); G. Taylor and J. Bishop (eds), *Being deaf: the experience of deafness* (London: Pinter Publishers, 1991); J.V. Van Cleve (ed.), *Deaf history unveiled* (Washington, DC: Gallaudet University Press, 1993) are just a few examples of this work

8   Hill, J. and J. Williams (eds), *Sport and identity in the north of England* (Keele: Keele University Press, 1996), p. 3

9   Holt, R., *Sport and the British* (Oxford: Oxford University Press, 1989) pp. 357–368

10   See, for example, Padden and Humphries, *Deaf in America*

11   Puttnam, R. D., *Bowling alone: the collapse and revival of American community* (New York: Simon and Schuster, 2000)

12   Anderson, B., *Imagined communities: reflections on the origin and spread of nationalism* (London: Verso, 1991)

13   Bale, J., *Sport, space and the city* (London: Routledge, 1993); Y-F. Tuan, *Topophilia: a study of environmental perception, attitudes and values* (London: Prentice-Hall, 1974); J.M. Wise, 'Home: territory and identity', *Cultural Studies* 14, 2 (2000), pp. 295–310

2

DEFINING THE DEAF COMMUNITY AND DEAF CULTURE IN BRITAIN

Public perceptions of deafness and deaf people have been (and remain) heavily influenced by medical views that promote the opinion that deaf people suffer from a condition that needs to be cured. This pathological perception of deaf people, reinforced by official acknowledgement of deafness as a disability, is indeed shared by many deaf people. It must be accepted that the majority of deaf people would prefer not to be so and view it is as a debilitating factor in their daily lives. However, for a small but significant proportion of the deaf population these negative perceptions are at odds with the way they see themselves. These deaf people see their deafness in much more positive terms and regard themselves as members of a vibrant deaf community, based on shared language and a common culture. As deaf clubs are seen as the homes of the deaf community and deaf culture, it is important to clarify what is meant by the terms 'deaf community' and 'deaf culture' as they are used within this book.

Various models have been constructed since the 1960s that attempt to determine who should be regarded as belonging to the deaf community, and what the cultural aspects of that community involve. These will be discussed in this chapter and the various criteria by which membership is determined will be outlined. However a closer examination of these theoretical models indicates that certain aspects do not sit easily with the reality of deaf life. This is especially true when the leisure activities of deaf people are assessed. These models will therefore be challenged in the light of the evidence of deaf people's shared leisure activities that will be presented in later chapters. In doing so, a case can be made for taking a much broader view of who actually constitutes the deaf community than is suggested by these models. A number of factors need to be considered as part of this discussion, including the ways in which deafness has historically been perceived in medical terms and deaf people portrayed as disabled; the way in which different groups of deaf people are differentiated from each other; the argument for the existence of a community of people based on their shared experiences of deafness; and the role of sign language in the cultural expression of the deaf community. The place of hearing people in the deaf community is a contentious issue that has stimulated much debate, and so this will also be addressed.

Deafness is often seen as a hidden condition, with deaf people not being as obvious as – for example – those who are blind or who have restricted mobility. Many deaf people are often only identified through the wearing of hearing aids, a lack of effective verbal communication when interacting with hearing people, or through the use of sign language.[1] Nevertheless, people with some degree of hearing loss or inability to hear form a significant percentage of the population. In 1998, Young, Ackerman and Kyle suggested that around 8.5 million people in Great Britain had some form of hearing loss.[2] Although there are no comparable figures available covering the period of this research, it is likely that the ratio of deafened people within the overall population (around one in seven) remained at least the same throughout the twentieth century. Indeed, the ratio may even have been higher before the introduction of new drugs to combat the effects of diseases such as meningitis, which was a major cause of deafness in the early years of the post-war period. What is obvious from these figures is that deafness affects a large proportion of the population and is by no means uncommon. The vast majority of deaf people are older people who have become progressively deaf as a natural part of the ageing process, although there are also a variety of medical reasons that can result in deafness occurring at any age. Most of these people will have spent their lives, prior to becoming deaf, acquiring and using English, both spoken and written, as their principal form of communication. They therefore continue to rely upon English-based communication methods, supplemented by the wearing of hearing aids and in many cases the acquisition (often subconsciously) of enhanced lip reading skills.

There are, however, a significant number of deaf people for whom spoken language is inappropriate as a communication method. From data collected in 1989, the British Deaf Association (BDA) estimated that there were approximately 62,500 people in England, Wales and Northern Ireland, and a further 7,000 in Scotland, who were deaf and whose first or preferred language was British Sign Language (BSL).[3] These figures confirmed earlier statistics quoted by Ballantyne and Martin, which showed a roughly similar distribution, whilst Young, Ackerman and Kyle cite similar figures more recently.[4] Although such figures are generally accepted, deafness is not a notifiable medical condition in Britain, and so there are no precise official records on the number of deaf sign language users at any particular time. The vast majority of these people are born deaf, or become deaf prior to acquiring spoken language skills (identified as 'pre-lingually deaf'), and as a result will not have a working knowledge of spoken or written English to the levels taken for granted by the hearing population.[5] A series of studies have confirmed that this group of deaf people belong to a distinct linguistic and cultural minority, certain aspects of whose lives differ significantly from the hearing majority as a direct result of their deafness.[6] This view is also shared by many deaf people who regard their deafness as part of their cultural makeup, and this issue is discussed in more detail below. Amongst the general population, comparatively little is known about this small section of the population, who use a visual-gestural form of communication from both choice and necessity, and a number of misconceptions have arisen about deafness and deaf people. For example, there seems to be a perception amongst much of the hearing population that all deaf people are expert lip-readers. This is not true, as deaf people have no greater innate ability to lip-read than hearing people. It is through a greater dependency on lip-reading for communication that deaf people generally develop these skills to a higher level. Even then, lip-reading is an inexact science, with only partial accuracy being achievable even in ideal circumstances.[7] Other misconceptions relate to the use of sign language, which is often seen as being either merely English communicated by the hands and eyes rather than the voice and ears, or alternatively as a loose collection of random gestures or mime.[8] Again, neither of these is true (although there are elements of mime and gesture inherent within sign language) with the pioneering work of Stokoe and many others since showing the linguistic and grammatical basis of signed languages.[9] After actually being deaf, sign language use is seen as the single most important defining characteristic necessary to belong to this cultural minority, representing the most appropriate medium through which the cultural life of the deaf community can be expressed and enjoyed.[10] In some respects, sign language use could be considered equally as important as deafness, as there is no minimum requirement for the degree of deafness or proficiency in sign language in order to be regarded as a member of the deaf community.

Deafness and disability

It is important to discuss the issue of whether deafness constitutes a disability, as this is a perception shared by many people outside the deaf world. Devas argues that impairment and disability arise from different causes.[11] In this perspective of disability, impairment is regarded as a physical condition or limitation, whilst disability is a form of social oppression that results from attitudes towards that impairment held by those who do not share it. Restrictions

resulting from impairment – such as the inability of a deaf person to communicate effectively in spoken English – are then blamed on the impaired person.
Most external conceptions of deafness refer to deaf people in medical or pathological terms, that is, as people who have a loss or an impairment which needs
to be cured or overcome, and this negative perception has profound impacts
on the way deaf people are dealt with by the hearing world.[12] This perception
has a very long history, Aristotle supposedly declaring 'those who are deaf are
also dumb', with the latter being subsequently interpreted as 'stupid' or 'incapable'. [13] This perception has largely held sway ever since, gaining strength from
its adaptation by religious groups and passing into various legal systems. The
Jewish Talmud, although acknowledging that deaf people had certain rights
(such as the right to have a marriage ceremony conducted in sign language),
denied them others, and both Greek and Roman law echoed this situation. In
turn, this perspective of deaf people passed into the canons of the Christian
Church, even finding expression in the Bible, and thus took hold in the perception of the wider population.[14] This negative image of deafness is still encountered by deaf people on a daily basis today, with the predominant perspective of
hearing people being 'a view that the principal characteristic of deafness is the
lack of something, i.e. hearing and/or communication ability'.[15] The response
of the hearing majority to this perceived lack has been to try to cure deafness
by making the deaf person as 'normal' as possible. This process of normalisa-
tion was pursued during the post-1945 period through a policy of education
based largely on the development of speech and lip reading ability, and the use
of technology such as ever smaller and more powerful hearing aids to achieve
this goal. Only those deaf people who managed to communicate effectively
in English were regarded as academically successful; the use of sign language
was only appropriate for those who were considered to be educational failures
through their inability to develop good speech and reading skills.[16]

Many people who are deaf share these negative perceptions of their deafness, particularly those who have become deafened after having lived as a
hearing person. In such cases, deafness can indeed represent a profound loss,
with many of those who become deafened considering themselves disabled
as a result.[17] Padden argued that those who are deafened prefer labels such as
'hard of hearing', which are seen more positively than 'deaf'.[18] For such deaf
people, who form the majority of the deaf element within the broader population, deafness does not contribute positively to their cultural identity. The term
'deaf community' generally refers only to the minority of deaf people for whom
being deaf is a celebrated part of their cultural identity. These deaf people view
themselves not in medical terms, but as members of a distinct cultural and
linguistic minority. The central identifier for culturally deaf people is the use

of sign language as their first or preferred method of communication, which is regarded as the most appropriate form of communication for profoundly deaf people. For this group of people, deafness per se is not seen as the disabling factor in their lives, and the notion of deafness as a disability is rejected, although they accept that they may be disabled as a result of widely held medical perceptions of deafness.[19] What they reject is the notion that this disability arises from deaf people themselves; instead, culturally deaf people echo Devas in considering that it is the attitude of the hearing majority towards deaf people that is the disabling factor.[20]

The lack of official recognition of sign language in Britain and any meaningful policy for the widespread use and availability of sign language in publicly funded primary and secondary education are seen as a central part of the disabling process. The rejection of sign language by the scientific community is – according to Kyle and Woll – very much a twentieth-century phenomenon. They cite earlier researchers who viewed the development of signed languages as following a natural linguistic pattern.[21] Sign languages were viewed as genuine – if primitive – forms of communication, sharing many of the linguistic features found in spoken languages. The later rejection of sign language as a true language (in linguistic and grammatical terms) resulted in the unique cultural identifier for deaf people also being rejected, and by extension the existence of a recognisable cultural and linguistic minority was denied. The non-recognition of British Sign Language as a native language of Britain, coupled with the continuing dominance of medical perceptions of deafness, is at the heart of the deafness as disability debate for many deaf people.[22] However, in circumstances where being considered 'disabled' can bring advantages, there is a marked ambivalence in the attitudes of some deaf people who otherwise reject the label. In Britain, deaf people are officially classified as disabled and are therefore entitled to specific State benefits. These include Disabled Living Allowance and Disabled Students Allowance. Many deaf people are happy to claim these benefits, and indeed fiercely defend their rights to do so, whilst at the same time rejecting any notion of deafness being a disability. Whether this attitude towards the material benefits of being considered disabled represents hypocrisy or pragmatism on the part of those deaf people claiming these benefits is not a matter for discussion here. In terms of whether deafness is regarded as a disability within the context of this book, my position is the following. The widely held view that deafness constitutes a disability is considered when it is appropriate or relevant to do so, and whilst it is acknowledged that deaf people are often disabled by society's perception of their deafness, deafness of itself does not constitute a disability.

The rejection of the concept of deafness as a disability is illustrated in the context of leisure and sport by the self-imposed isolation of deaf sport from the

International Paralympic Movement. The Comite Internationale des Sports des Sourds (CISS) was formed as the governing body for international deaf sport in 1924, and founded the Silent Games in the same year as the deaf version of the Olympic Games. The Silent Games were renamed the Deaf Olympiad in 1949, and the CISS joined the International Olympic Movement in 1951. In consequence, the title was changed to World Games for the Deaf and CISS was recognised by the International Olympic Committee as an 'international federation of Olympic standing'. CISS formally joined the Paralympic Olympic Committee in 1988, with the World Games for the Deaf being recognised as having the same status as the Paralympics. As part of the agreement, CISS was to receive a percentage of the funding available to disabled sport provided through the Paralympic Olympic Committee. The growing debate over the status of deafness as a disability and its implications for deaf sport led to the withdrawal of CISS from the Paralympic Olympic Committee in 1995. Other disabled sports groups had started to query the special status awarded to deaf athletes in being allowed to hold their own separate games, and demands were made for deaf athletes to be included in the Paralympics. Rather than agree to integration under the umbrella of disabled sport, CISS withdrew, losing the funding provided through the Paralympic Olympic Committee in the process. The perception of deafness as a disability was rejected by the deaf sporting community, despite the severe financial implications for all levels of deaf sport that resulted from adopting such a stance. In 2001, a rapprochement was achieved when the World Games for the Deaf was rebranded 'Deaflympics', and the summer and winter events are now sanctioned by the International Olympic Committee.[23]

The notion of 'the deaf community'

The academic concept of a 'deaf community' arose as a direct result of the work of William Stokoe in the 1950s and early 1960s, who identified linguistic features of American Sign Language (ASL) that clearly showed that ASL was a true language, and not merely a collection of randomly generated gestures.[24] The *Dictionary of American Sign Language* also attempted to illustrate the ways in which sign language use affects and influences the social and cultural characteristics of deaf people.[25] Since this pioneering work, there has been a great deal of academic discussion on the composition and membership of what has come to be termed 'the deaf community'. Stokoe's work was taken up in Britain by academics such as Brennan, Colville and Lawson and Woll, Kyle and Deuchar, who found similar results when researching the linguistics of British Sign Language (BSL).[26] Through the academic recognition of signed languages as true languages, the languages came to be seen as the means of cultural expression and identification for and by their users:

> ... the discussion of the 'linguistic community' of Deaf people in the *Dictionary of ASL* represented a break from the long tradition of pathologizing Deaf people. In a sense the book brought official and public recognition of a deeper aspect of Deaf people's lives: their culture.[27]

The argument followed that if a group of people shared a common language and a common culture, then they naturally formed a community, and this has largely been accepted, although medical perceptions of deafness and deaf people continue to be huge influential amongst the general public.

The existence of a deaf community in Britain (and elsewhere) is accepted by those involved with the deaf world, and has been the basis of an increasing body of research since the 1970s. Whilst this research may have introduced the concept of a deaf community, the reality of a community of like-minded people gathering together and sharing their experiences and interests does not stem from this period. It was not the academic recognition of sign language that resulted in the formation of the deaf community: the community was already there, if largely unrecognised and unacknowledged by wider society. There is extensive evidence from the pages of the deaf print media, such as the *British Deaf News* and its predecessors, which clearly shows that a deaf community has existed in Britain for many years; in fact ever since deaf people in England began to gather together in the deaf schools established from the early nineteenth century.[28]

Although the deaf community as an entity has existed for a considerable time, the term 'deaf community' only appeared in Britain from around 1980. A collection of papers published by the National Union of the Deaf over the period 1976 to 1986 offers an insight into the development of the use of the term by deaf writers themselves.[29] *Deaf Liberation* includes a variety of terms to describe the deaf element of the population, with 'deaf people' being by far the most commonly used until around 1980, but there were several others which appeared regularly such as 'the deaf' and 'the deaf world'. Some older writers even persisted with the use of 'deaf and dumb' and 'deaf mute', both terms that are now regarded as demeaning and unacceptable.[30] From around 1980 onwards, the term 'deaf community' was used much more regularly, but not exclusively. Perhaps significantly, this was the start of increased political activity amongst deaf sign language users, and the term and the concept of 'deaf community' seem to have developed symbiotically. 'Deaf community' has remained the term of choice and the standard way of describing the group identity of this particular group of deaf people ever since. The subsequent evolution of the concepts of 'Deaf Nation' and 'Deaf World' in recent years is discussed later in this chapter, but these are based very much within the wider context of 'the deaf community'.

The major difference between the deaf community and other minority communities is that deaf people do not have an obvious geographical focus; there is no area of a town or country where deaf people group together to live in the way that other communities do. Deaf people generally live in isolation from each other in their daily lives, except for members of their family who may also be deaf. One reason for this is that the vast majority of deaf people are born into hearing families with two hearing parents; nor do deaf parents necessarily have deaf children, particularly if one or both parents have become deafened through illness or injury rather than for any genetic reason.[31] Instead of living together in geographical communities, deaf people have found alternative ways of coming together, with residential deaf schools and the extensive network of deaf social clubs around Britain playing a vital role in bringing deaf people together and introducing younger deaf people to the life and culture of the community. This gathering together of people from similar audiological and experiential backgrounds took place mostly within the network of deaf clubs that grew up in virtually every large town and city in Britain during the nineteenth and twentieth centuries. As Kyle and Woll assert, 'the central environments for deaf interaction are the social clubs which exist throughout the UK'.[32] Even when coming together as a community of like-minded people with similar outlooks and life experiences, deaf people as a community remained largely isolated, but in this case by choice. In many ways, it is this coming together within a world of their own creation that serves as the second major defining characteristic of the deaf community after sign language use.[33] As Padden points out: 'Deaf people had long recognized that their groups are different from those of hearing people'. Deaf clubs provided the venues for this difference to find expression and celebration, rather than being seen as a disability or handicap.[34] Deaf newspapers contained details of the wide range of activities that deaf people participated in, both as individuals and most importantly as groups. Deaf club members had a varied social life that brought an essentially isolated collection of individuals together in a way that conformed to various definitions of a community, as will be illustrated in later chapters.

The academic argument for the existence of the deaf community is now widely accepted, but defining the deaf community has exercised writers on deaf issues for a number of years. Several models have been constructed which attempt to define the criteria for membership, by identifying ways in which acceptance into the community can be achieved. These remain in use today whenever the deaf community is discussed in academic contexts and have become the accepted standards by which membership is determined. However, by attempting to set out strict rules for membership, it is often easier to identify those who do not belong than to be sure who is definitely a member. By being so prescriptive, these models only make the situation more confusing and the various arguments regarding membership are less valid as a result. This is not to claim that these models are necessarily wrong, but evidence presented later in this study will support the argument that the narrow criteria outlined in some of these models does not fully reflect the reality of deaf life. In addition, none of these models are based on empirical historical evidence. When the history of leisure activity amongst deaf club members is investigated, the deaf community is found to have been much less restrictive or restricted than the models and their associated criteria suggest.

Deaf or deaf?

In order to distinguish between the two supposedly distinct groups of deaf people, a convention was adopted in the early 1970s which involves the use of capital and lower case 'D' when writing the word 'deaf'.[35] 'Deaf' is used when referring to those people who regard their deafness as a culturally defining factor in their identity – the group generally referred to as 'the deaf community'. This group includes those deaf people whose first or preferred language is sign language. The word 'deaf' is used for those people whose deafness is merely an audiological condition, rather than having any linguistic or cultural connotations. This group includes those people who refer to themselves as 'deafened', 'hard of hearing', 'hearing impaired' and similar labels. This convention has been generally accepted and used amongst the majority of writers on the deaf community as the means by which membership of the deaf community is acknowledged or denied. However, this convention is both unhelpful and confusing, as in practice, 'Deaf' has often come to be used as a means of exclusion rather than inclusion. The lower case 'd' is often used in pejorative terms, indicating those who are considered to be of inferior status as deaf people. An Orwellian 'Big D good, little d bad' is often a hidden subtext of the allocation of these labels, as shown by the use of 'RNId' amongst politically active deaf sign language users. The argument is that the Royal National Institute for Deaf People (RNID) does not reflect the wishes and aspirations of sign language users and only works on behalf of those deaf people who are not members of the deaf community. Therefore, the use of a capital D in their acronym is rejected by the more politically active members of the deaf community.

In a reappraisal of who belongs in the deaf community, Lawson states that those who might be seen as 'deaf' (i.e. not culturally deaf) historically had a place within the deaf community. The concept of 'Deaf' and 'deaf' has left many such people feeling excluded and hurt by the attitudes of those they regarded as fellow deaf people. As Lawson points out, these deaf people played an active part in the community and suffered the same prejudice and treatment by the hearing majority as deaf people who used sign language. [36] Padden and Humphries attempted to deal with the issues that arise by declaring that 'Deaf people are both Deaf and deaf'.[37] This may be true within the parameters suggested by Woodward, but this statement does nothing to address the confusion that arises through the use of d/D. To try to resolve this dichotomy, some authors adopted 'D/deaf', both to avoid assigning an unwarranted status to individual deaf people and to encompass all deaf people whether 'Deaf' or 'deaf'. The convention is gradually disappearing from academic works on deafness and deaf people but can still be found in use. For the above reasons, and in order to avoid the potential confusions outlined earlier, the lower case 'd' in deaf is used throughout this book as an umbrella term to reflect the experiences of deaf individuals and groups. The lower case is intended to be inclusive and it is used consistently for all references to deafness, deaf people and deaf community in the text. However, in quotations the usage of the original text has been retained.

Attempting to differentiate between those who 'belong' and those who do not led to various criteria being proposed to determine membership of the deaf community, but these models do not address many of the questions that arise as a result. Writing in 1980, Higgins argued that whilst deafness is 'a necessary condition', deafness alone is not sufficient to warrant membership of the deaf community, and other writers support this position. He contended that membership cannot be assumed, but must be conferred by existing community members, or achieved through 'identification with the deaf world; shared experiences that come from being deaf; and participation in the community's activities'. [38] The underlying problem with this model is that it does not allow for the inclusion of hearing people in the deaf community. Indeed, Higgins clearly states that 'hearing people are not part of the deaf community'.[39] Lawson also made no allowance for the inclusion of hearing people, when she described the British deaf community as being 'the deaf "in group"'. [40] Despite the claims of Higgins and Lawson, hearing people have always been accepted into the deaf community, whilst participation in the community's activities has long been a part of the social life of hearing children of deaf parents. In doing so, they gained some measure of identification with the deaf world simply through association with deaf people. Although not deaf themselves, hearing family members deal with the consequences of deafness on a daily basis and so share the overall experience of being deaf to a large extent. Without displaying the correct attitude, it is unlikely that hearing people would be accepted into the social life of the deaf community, and the evidence shows that they were involved in the activities of the deaf clubs. Therefore, to say that hearing people cannot be part of the deaf community does not fully reflect the true situation. In his version of the deaf community, Ladd agreed with Higgins and Lawson that the sharing of cultural values is an essential requirement for membership.[41] However, he took a more realistic view by making allowance for the inclusion of hearing people, on the basis that the deaf person may have hearing family, friends and acquaintances who support and are involved in the cultural life of the deaf community.

Baker-Shenk and Cokely defined four routes of entry by which membership of the deaf community can be achieved: audiological; political; linguistic; social.[42] The only route not open to hearing people is that of being deaf. However, Baker-Shenk and Cokely argue that in order to be a full or 'core' member, involved in the very heart of the deaf community and its culture, all four criteria need to be met in combination with the necessary positive attitude. This implies that only deaf sign language users can be fully immersed in the cultural life of the deaf community, as only they can have access via all four routes. However, this model does relate more closely to the experiences of both deaf and hearing community members. Padden also accepted the place of hearing people within the deaf community, but made a similar distinction between those who are community members and those who are actively involved in deaf culture. She argued that access to deaf culture is more closed than gaining access to the deaf community, and only those who are deaf can fully participate in deaf culture. Padden defined the culturally deaf core of the deaf community as those who:

> behave as Deaf people do, use the language of Deaf people and share the beliefs that Deaf people have about themselves and those who are not Deaf.[43]

As Padden pointed out, the cultural life of the deaf community requires evidence of certain behaviour and attitudes. However, people who are not deaf can meet the criteria for core membership if they are involved in the social life of a deaf club. When in the deaf clubs, hearing people have to use sign language in order to communicate and participate fully; through interacting with deaf people, they are to a large extent acting as deaf people do; by choosing to take part, they are sharing the beliefs of deaf people. Three of the avenues for membership outlined by Baker-Shenk and Cokely are thus available to those who are not deaf and so the final requirement (to be deaf) is called into question. If someone is socially, politically and linguistically active within the deaf community, then it would seem that they are deeply immersed in all aspects of the community's shared life and culture, whether they are deaf or hearing.

One requirement that is almost totally absent from the various attempts to define the deaf community is for a minimum level of deafness. Anyone who is deaf – to whatever degree – can become a member of the deaf community, even the cultural core included in several models. Padden and Markowitz concluded that 'audiometric deafness, the actual degree of hearing loss, often has little to do with where a person relates in the Deaf community'.[44] Padden further clarified the necessary level of deafness in order to be considered 'Deaf':

> the type or degree of hearing loss is not a criterion for being Deaf. Rather, the criterion is whether a person identifies with other Deaf people, or behaves as a Deaf person.[45]

Higgins is the only author to suggest that a minimum level of deafness is required in order to qualify for community membership. In doing so, he provides further grounds for re-examining the question of who should be considered as a member of the deaf community. Higgins argued that children whom he classed as hard of hearing (rather than deaf) often became members of the deaf community as a result of misdiagnosis of their degree of deafness.[46] Because they were placed in what Higgins considered to be the 'inappropriate setting' of deaf schools, these children effectively learned how to be deaf. This came from mixing socially with deaf children and developing patterns of behaviour normally associated with profoundly deaf people, such as sign language use. He concluded that these children were only 'socially deaf' rather than being sufficiently 'audiologically deaf' to warrant membership of the deaf community.[47] If such people can learn how to 'behave as deaf people do' through shared social activity and acquired behaviour, then hearing people must surely be able to find acceptance in the same manner. The evidence of deaf club activity indicates that in fact hearing people have always been accepted into the social life of the community, notwithstanding their lack of deafness.

There have been several instances of people with a lesser degree of hearing impairment, or who became deafened later in life, becoming respected members of the deaf community.[48] Some of these have even attained the status of members of the cultural centre of the community, as defined by Padden and Baker-Shenk and Cokely.[49] Padden states that for those who come to the deaf community later in life, there are often conflicts between the values and perspectives learnt from living in the hearing world and those held by the deaf community. It is only those who accept the views of the deaf community who are successfully integrated into the deaf world.[50] Those who feel themselves to be part of the deaf community because of shared deafness and having positive attitudes towards their deafness would thus appear to be members. However, it is also argued that membership has to be conferred, not assumed. Evidence of the social activities of deaf people presented later indicates that deaf people have been much more pragmatic about conferring community membership than the theoretical models would suggest. Several deaf clubs had 'hard of hearing' sections for those deaf people who did not use sign language, for example. Similarly, hearing people are mentioned in reports of deaf club activity on a regular basis. Such evidence shows that the various criteria for membership outlined in the academic models were less rigidly applied in the everyday life of deaf clubs and the deaf community. Indeed, writing as early as 1988, Paddy Ladd proposed that 'British sign language community' should replace 'British deaf community' in order to acknowledge that use of and respect for BSL was the key admission criteria rather than an individual's audiological status.[51]

Despite these apparent weaknesses, the various models described above remain the standard academic and theoretical means by which membership is determined. There have been no radical attempts to redefine the criteria for membership since the mid-1980s, and these models have not been fundamentally challenged in any way. Much of the subsequent discussion has centred more on whether the deaf community should be viewed as an ethnic group, because of the linguistic aspect of membership.[52] This view of deafness led to much discussion of the concept of 'the Deaf Nation' towards the end of the twentieth century and more recently 'Deafhood' was proposed as the next stage of development, although this has not been widely adopted as an aspect of daily deaf life.[53] The prospect of a 'Deaf Nation' emerging – at least as an ideological concept if not a geographical reality – is not an impossibility. Many of the factors identified by Anderson in the development of nation states based on 'imagined communities' can be found in the evolution of the deaf community into a 'Deaf Nation'.[54] These include a sense of shared oppression; knowledge of the language of the 'pre-nation' community as an essential to gaining membership; the decline in the importance of religion in daily life; and even the role of newspapers as 'cultural product'.[55]

Amongst these later developments, the concept and definition of 'deaf community' seems to have been quietly dropped as a topic for discussion:

> It is interesting that the discussion has shifted from 'Deaf Community' to 'Deaf Nation' at a time when most Deaf people are just about grasping the meaning of 'Deaf Community'. Many Deaf people are still only paying lip service to 'Deaf Culture and Deaf Community' without being too sure what they actually mean.[56]

As this quotation from Alker suggests, many deaf people do not fully grasp what the term 'deaf community' really means. This supports the argument that there remains some distance between the narrow views on membership based on academic criteria and the practical realities of everyday deaf life.

The culture of the deaf community

Although many markers and forms of behaviour exhibited by deaf people have been identified as examples of deaf culture, the validity of some of these supposedly unique deaf cultural activities might be questioned. An often-quoted statistic is that 90 to 95 per cent of deaf people marry other deaf people, but it is highly likely that this ratio is also true of many other cultural minority groups.[57] Lane, Hofmeister and Bahan argue that the deaf community frown upon marriage between deaf and hearing people; Higgins claims that having a deaf spouse does not guarantee a hearing person acceptance into the deaf community.[58] Again, the same could be said to apply to many minorities. Whilst these statements might have some basis in reality, it is more likely that the communication difficulties between deaf sign language users and potential hearing partners are a more effective barrier than peer pressure. Indeed, when communication between deaf and hearing people is not an issue, relationships can and do form, as shown by the number of such relationships that occur amongst students at the University of Central Lancashire.[59] Hearing students reading for a degree in Deaf Studies learn sign language as part of their course, and the university also attracts a large number of signing deaf students for a variety of courses. In this setting, relationships between deaf and hearing occur regularly and naturally as the communication barrier is removed.

Rather than being prescriptive in determining what constitutes deaf culture, it is more reflective of the life of the deaf community to consider deaf culture as those activities and behaviours deaf people share when they gather together. There are no doubt some similarities with the cultural lives of hearing people, and the main defining element of deaf culture is the medium of expression used – sign language. However, speech and sound can play a part in the cultural and social lives of deaf people. For example, some deaf people choose to speak when they sign, or to vary their method of communication depending on whom they are communicating with. Some deaf people choose to speak to each other rather than use sign in certain settings, but despite this, some writers have argued that speech has no place in deaf culture.[60] Evidence will also be presented which shows that sound-based activities play an important role in the social lives of deaf people. To say that something a deaf person freely chooses to do is not part of their culture seems to be the arbitrary application of personal biases onto others. Using speech is a part of the everyday lives of many deaf people, and often arises as a pragmatic solution to the situation they find themselves in. Unlike the use of technology (such as flashing door bells), this is a pattern of behaviour that arises directly from deaf life. As Padden and Humphries point out: '[The deaf community] have found ways to define and express themselves through their rituals, tales, performances and everyday social encounters'. [61] In other words, through the types of activities that take place naturally whenever deaf people come together, whether this is in deaf clubs or elsewhere. It seems unnecessary to try and define what is or is not a part of that culture any more precisely than this. Whilst there are some defining characteristics, such as the use of sign language, it is argued here that anything can become a part of deaf culture if it is something deaf people do – or choose to do – as part of their patterns of behaviour. As the analysis of deaf leisure activity will show, deaf people often choose – of their own free will – to engage in certain activities and in a certain way that do not fit within the generally accepted theories and boundaries of 'deaf culture'. Therefore, it is argued that the element of choice means these activities should be considered as part of deaf cultural activity, whatever they may be.

A community of deaf people, who indulge in a range of activities with other deaf people, and whose patterns of social behaviour are, in some ways, dictated by their deafness, most certainly exists. However, some of the definitions of the deaf community posited by various academics include criteria for member-ship that will be contradicted by the evidence of deaf leisure activities which appears in later chapters. For the purposes of this book, the deaf community is defined as those people whose deafness gives rise to interests and experiences that they actively share and participate in with other deaf people. This group can include both people who were born deaf and those who have become deafened at some stage in their life. The use of sign language as the primary or preferred method of communication is a central feature of the social life of the deaf community and its members and is therefore a defining element in identifying the focus group for this research. However, this need not exclude those who in various parts of their lives also use speech and lip-reading through choice or necessity. The main method of determining who are members of the deaf community is that these are primarily deaf people, who take part in the activities of a deaf club, and in which setting they choose to share their leisure time and interests with other members.

There still remains the issue of the place of hearing people within the deaf community, and whether or not they can be members. Deaf people live, mix and co-exist within a hearing majority, and this extends to certain aspects of their personal and social lives. As evidence produced later will show, hearing people – such as spouses, relatives and friends – have always played an active role in the social life of the deaf community. By accepting hearing people into their community and its leisure activities, membership of the deaf commu-nity was at least partially or temporarily conferred. By extension, these hear-ing people were involved in the cultural life of the deaf community, and so must have had some impact and input into deaf culture; they were not merely passive observers of deaf culture taking place. In the reports of deaf club activity, there was often little indication of the audiological status of those taking part, and so participation in any particular event may have included members who were sign language users, deafened or hard of hearing, or even hearing. Therefore, it is not possible to say with any certainty whether an event was attended solely by deaf or sign language using members. As the reports of deaf club life used for this research give no indication of different levels of deafness amongst members or whether hearing members were involved, no differentiation is considered necessary. Indeed, given the lack of available evidence, no such differentiation is practicable or achievable. The sole criterion will be that it was an activity engaged in by deaf club members and therefore part of the culture of the particular deaf club, no matter who was involved.

The deaf community and its particular culture are not entirely different from those of the hearing world, although certain elements of deaf life may be. Previous investigations into deaf community life and deaf culture have suggested that deaf people view the world and act in a totally different way to their hearing neighbours. The evidence of deaf club activity shows that whilst it might be argued that deaf people have a different perception of the world, they have not taken part in any leisure activities that are markedly different from their hearing neighbours. Therefore, deaf culture is defined as those activities deaf people chose to take part in when they gathered together and the patterns of behaviour they demonstrated in such situations. Leisure and sport have played an important role in bringing deaf people together, and in doing so helped to create and maintain a community based on shared experiences of deafness. It is for this reason that this research focuses on the activities of deaf club members. As will be shown in the following chapter, it is generally agreed that deaf clubs have served as the centre of deaf cultural life. Therefore it follows that the activities of these members constituted a major part of that culture.

In order to justify taking such a broad view of deaf culture, this book illustrates not only the raw details of the leisure and sporting activities of deaf club members, but also the way these activities served to bring and bond deaf people together. As has been shown, the deaf community is based on shared experiences, a shared social life and the communal identity that directly results from shared deafness. However, none of the models outlined earlier relate theoretical notions of either the deaf community or deaf culture to empirical historical evidence to support the positions taken. The detailed investigation of deaf club members' leisure and sporting interests presented here for the first time shows that these activities served as an important form of communal cultural expression. When deaf leisure and sport are investigated closely, the results show how deaf people used these shared activities as more than just a way of passing their spare time. This sharing of leisure time helped deaf club members to find group and self-identity within a community of people with similar experiences and world views. This investigation shows that the views of what constitutes 'deaf culture' are somewhat narrow and not fully representative of the range of deaf people's individual and communal leisure practices. By showing precisely what deaf people have chosen to do in their spare time, with whom and in which settings, the broader view of deaf culture proposed here will be seen to be entirely justified, as this reflects the reality of deaf life much more accurately than the theoretical concepts of 'deaf community' and 'deaf culture'. Padden defined those at the cultural core of the deaf community as 'behaving as deaf people do'; this research will show exactly what 'behaving as deaf people do' involved in post-war Britain. [62]

In using these parameters to define both deaf people and deaf culture, the intention is to include all those who regard themselves as actively involved in the leisure life of the deaf community. By focusing on deaf club members, the experiences of a wide range of deaf people are accurately reflected, and the variety of activities and perspectives that fall under the generic labels of 'the deaf community' and 'deaf culture' are represented. It is these people and their activities that form the focus for this research, without any preconditions being applied to determine whether they fit precisely any of the models for membership of the deaf community outlined above. Having established and defined both the deaf community and deaf culture as they are understood within the context of this study, it is necessary to show how this geographically dispersed collection of individuals came to form a distinct and identifiable body of people.

Notes

1   Woolley, M., 'Signs of strife – signs of life' in Lee, *Deaf liberation*, pp. 85–91

2   Young, A., J. Ackerman and J. Kyle, *Looking on: deaf people and the organisation of services* (Bristol: Polity Press, 1998), p. 1

3   British Deaf Association website: www.britishdeafassociation.org.uk/bsl/page

4   Ballantyne, J. and J.A.M. Martin, *Deafness* (Edinburgh: Livingstone, 1984) pp. 1–2; Young *et al.*, *Looking on*, p.1

5   Brennan, M., *Word formation in British Sign Language* (Stockholm: University of Stockholm, 1990); J. Anderson, *Deaf student mis-writing, teacher mis-reading: English education and the deaf college student* (Burtonsville: Linstok, 1993), pp. 12–52

6   These include Baker-Shenk and Padden, *American Sign Language*; Kyle and Woll, *Sign language*; Padden and Humphries, *Deaf in America*; Sutton-Spence and Woll, *The linguistics of British Sign Language*

7   Royal National Institution for Deaf People, *Watch this face: a practical guide to lipreading* (London: RNID, 2002)

8   Kyle and Woll, *Sign language* pp. 24–57

9   See for example W.C. Stokoe, D.C. Casteline and C.G. Croneberg, *A dictionary of American Sign Language on linguistic principles* (Silver Spring: Linstok Press, 1965); W.C. Stokoe, 'Sign language structure: an outline of the visual communication system of the American deaf', *Studies in Linguistics* (New York: Academic Press, 1960)

10   Ladd, 'The modern deaf community' pp. 37–38

11   Devas, M. 'Support and access in sports and leisure provision', *Disability and Society* 18, 2 (2003), pp. 231–245

12   Kyle and Woll, *Sign language*, pp. 6–7; H. Lane, R. Hofmeister and B. Bahan, *A journey into the DEAF-WORLD* (San Diego: DawnSignPress, 1996), pp. 365–366

13   Higgins, *Outsiders*, p.24; M.G. McLoughlin, *A history of the education of the deaf in England* (Gosport: Ashford Colour Press, 1987), pp. 1–2

14   See St Mark's Gospel, chapter 7, verses 31–37

15   Kyle and Woll, *Sign language*, p. 6

16   Conrad, R. 'Towards a definition of oral success' in Lee, *Deaf liberation*, pp. 27–32; W. Lynas, 'Integrating the handicapped into ordinary schools' in Gregory and Hartley, *Constructing* deafness, pp. 151–156

17   Wright, D., *Deafness: a personal account* (London: Allen Lane, 1969); Woolley, 'Signs of strife'

18   Padden, C., 'The deaf community and deaf culture' in Gregory and Hartley *Constructing deafness*, p. 44

19   Corker, *Deaf and disabled*

20   Finkelstein, 'We are not disabled'; H. Lane, 'Do Deaf people have a disability?' — address given to the Federation of Deaf People conference, Blackburn, 7 November 1998

21   Kyle and Woll, *Sign language* pp. 46–48

22   The British Government finally recognised BSL as a true language in 2003, but the language still has no official status as a native language in Britain

23   www.deaflympics.com

24   Stokoe, 'Sign language structure'

25   Stokoe *et al.*, *A dictionary of American Sign Language*

26   Brennan, M., M. Colville and L. Lawson, *Words in hand: a structural analysis of the signs of British Sign Language* (Edinburgh: Moray House College of Education, 1980); B. Woll, J. Kyle and M. Deuchar (eds), *Perspectives on British Sign Language and deafness* (London: Croom Helm, 1981)

27   Padden, 'The deaf community and deaf culture' p. 2

28   Lawson, 'The role of sign', p. 32

29   Lee, *Deaf liberation*

30   Finkelstein, 'We are not disabled', p. 266

31   The incidence of a deaf child having two hearing parents is as high as 90 to 95 per cent according to Lane *et al.*, *A journey into the DEAF-WORLD*, p. 30

32   Kyle and Woll, *Sign language*, p. 10

33   *Ibid.*, pp. 9–12

34   Padden, 'The deaf community and deaf culture', p. 2

35   Woodward, J.C. 'Implications for sociolinguistic research amongst the deaf', *Sign Language Studies* 1 (1972), pp. 1–7

36   Lawson, L., 'Do we want one or multiple deaf nations?', *Deaf Worlds* 18, 3 (2002) pp. 96–102

37   Padden and Humphries, *Deaf in America*, p. 3

38   Higgins, *Outsiders*, p. 38

39   *Ibid.*, pp. 44–45

40   Lawson, 'The role of sign', p. 31

41   Ladd, 'The modern deaf community', p. 37–38

42   Baker-Shenk and Cokely *American Sign Language*, pp. 17–20

43   Padden, 'The deaf community and deaf culture', p. 44

44   Cited by J.C. Woodward, 'How you gonna get to heaven if you can't talk with Jesus?' in S. Wilcox (ed.), *American deaf culture* (Burtonsville: Linstock, 1989), p. 164

45   Padden, 'The deaf community and the culture of deaf people', p.8

46   Higgins, *Outsiders*, pp. 26–27

47   *Ibid.*, p. 44

48   Examples of such people include Lord Ashley and Maggie Woolley, as described in J. Ashley, *Acts of defiance* (London: Reinhardt, 1992) and Woolley, 'Signs of strife'

49   Padden, 'The deaf community and deaf culture', pp. 40–45; Baker-Shenk and Cokely, *American Sign Language*, pp. 17–20

50   Padden, 'The deaf community and deaf culture', p. 43

51   Ladd, 'The modern deaf community' pp. 37–38

52   Examples of this debate are given in Padden and Humphreys, *Deaf in America*, pp. 112–114; L.J. Davis, *Enforcing normalcy: disability, deafness and the body* (London: Verso, 1995), pp. 73–99

53   Alker, D., 'The realities of nationhood', *Deaf Worlds* 18, 3 (2002), pp. 79–82; S.D Emery, 'The Deaf Nation, five years on', *Deaf Worlds* 18, 2 (2002), pp. 103–104; P. Ladd, 'Emboldening the deaf nation', *Deaf Worlds* 18, 3 (2002), pp. 88–95; Lawson, 'Do we want one or multiple deaf nations?'; G.H. Turner, 'The deaf nation notion: citizenship, control and courage', *Deaf Worlds* 18, 3 (2002), pp. 74–78; Ladd, *Understanding deaf culture*

54   Anderson, *Imagined communities*

55   *Ibid.*, pp. 39–40

56   Alker, 'The realities of nationhood', p. 79

57   Lane *et al.*, *A journey into the DEAF-WORLD*, p. 71

58   *Ibid.*, p. 71; Higgins, *Outsiders*, p. 28

59   The author is Course Leader for Deaf Studies at the University of Central Lancashire, Preston, UK

60   For example, Padden, 'The deaf community and deaf culture', p. 42

61   Padden and Humphries, *Deaf in America*, p. 10

62   Padden, 'The deaf community and deaf culture', p. 44

3

THE DEVELOPMENT OF DEAF CLUBS
IN BRITAIN

The deaf community could not have come into existence without shared locations where socially isolated deaf people could gather and develop relationships based on common experiences and characteristics. As the previous chapter illustrated, deaf clubs have long been seen as the hub of deaf community life but little has been previously known about how or why they emerged other than that these deaf clubs arose from a number of local voluntary organisations set up to assist deaf people in their daily lives. In this chapter, the development of the deaf welfare organisations that emerged from the nineteenth century onwards is examined, and set within the wider context of welfare provision during the Victorian era. Examples of the types of people deemed worthy of charitable help and support highlight the way in which voluntary welfare bodies for deaf people emerged alongside those of other disadvantaged sections of the population. One of the main contentions of this chapter is that the 1834 Poor Law Amendment Act had a causal effect on the establishment of deaf welfare organisations, by placing deaf paupers in a contested position in terms of their suitability for support from the Poor Law Commissioners. Despite this legislation making no specific provision for impoverished deaf people, there were wide-reaching and long-lasting consequences for the deaf population of Britain which contributed to the establishment of a recognisable deaf community.

Deaf welfare formed just one part of a general trend to care for those seen to be disadvantaged within society that emerged during the nineteenth century, but the changes in the Poor Law acted as a major stimulus to the formation of deaf societies and independent welfare organisations. Evidence drawn from contemporary sources shows that deaf paupers were often placed in the workhouses, where they found themselves suffering all that the forbidding system entailed. As a consequence, various philanthropic measures were introduced to try to ensure as many deaf people as possible avoided this fate. Deaf socie-ties played a number of roles in this endeavour, such as providing vocational training and finding jobs for deaf people, but they also had a social function. By bringing deaf people together, the deaf clubs came to symbolise the social arms of these welfare societies and went on to play an integral part in bonding deaf people together as a community. Without the deaf clubs, the deaf commu-nity would have had no geographical focus and deaf people would have had nowhere to come together to socialise and enjoy a range of leisure and sporting activities. From a personal perspective, it is hard to see how else the modern deaf community could have come into existence if these clubs and societies had not emerged.

The Poor Law in England

It is not the intention here to provide a detailed analysis of poor law provi-sion and welfare development in Britain during the eighteenth and nine-teenth centuries. However, some background information is necessary in order to provide a contextual framework for the ways in which responses to the 1834 Poor Law Amendment Act influenced the emergence of volun-tary welfare bodies for deaf people and I am particularly indebted to Anne Borsay and Steven King for their work on this legislation.[1] Attitudes towards the poor hardened during the late eighteenth and early nineteenth centuries, as the growing urban populations overwhelmed the existing system of poor relief that dated back to 1601 and which was largely geared to responding to the cyclical effects of a predominantly agricultural economy. Under the 1601 Act, which formalised a series of earlier measures into one coherent system, parishes were obliged to provide poor relief for paupers in their area through Poor Law Boards made up of local ratepayers. Support in the form of parish doles was only to be provided for the 'deserving poor' – the old, infirm, widows and children – and would take the form of 'outdoor relief'. This allowed for the provision of money or goods whilst those receiving support continued to live in their own homes. The parish found employment for those without work, whilst those who designated 'able-bodied' but who refused to work were to be refused relief and punished for their indolence. Communal relief, through residence in a workhouse, was to be the last resort, only to be considered when all other means of supporting paupers had been exhausted. Various reforms and amendments to the poor law were introduced over the next two centu-ries, but two Acts in particular influenced the way in which poor relief was administered and provided. Knatchbull's Act of 1722/23 introduced the first formal workhouse test and established a system of relief for the able-bodied poor that required claimants to reside in the workhouse and provide work in return for shelter and food. In doing so, workhouses became the *de facto* venues for administering punishment – in the form of compulsory labour – on the indolent and undeserving poor, as had been a function of the Poor Law Boards since 1601. Gilbert's Act of 1782 sought to change the purpose of workhouses from centres of punishment to centres of care, by restricting admission to the impotent and therefore deserving poor. All others were to be eligible only for outdoor relief, but both Acts were only enabling measures; they did not impose or compel claimants of poor relief or the Poor Law Boards to follow these practices but merely provided a framework for those who chose to adopt them. [2]

Increased industrialisation, expanding urban environments and a series of trade depressions brought increased pressure on the system of poor relief as the eighteenth century ended and the nineteenth century began. The increasingly popular view amongst those administering – and most importantly paying for – the existing Poor Law provision was that the system was too permissive and so discouraged self-help and self-sufficiency by providing relief for all, whether they were capable of working or not. As a result, the old system of parish-based relief was reformed in 1834 and a more rigidly defined and centrally controlled regime was introduced. [3] The New Poor Law was intended to reduce the numbers claiming poor relief to all but the most desperate, through strict application of the principle of 'less eligibility'. Following this approach, life in the workhouse was intended to be nothing more than an unattractive and undesirable alternative to taking any work, no matter how poorly paid. In the workhouse husbands and wives were separated, with socialisation commonly limited to brief periods on Sundays, and there was a strict timetable involving ten hours of work in a day that typically began at five o'clock in the morning and ended with bed at eight o'clock in the evening. [4] Those who were deemed able to work had to perform various tasks in return for their upkeep, which was provided at a level that was less than the lowest locally available wage.

The 1834 Poor Law Amendment Act also brought in a much stricter application of the rules for determining who could claim relief, and in many respects, the New Poor Law (as it became known) saw a return to the principles established by the Knatchbull Act. The workhouses once more became places of punishment and deterrence for the indolent poor but in many instances, all claimants were forced to enter the workhouse, whether deserving or undeserving. Determining whether or not someone was 'able-bodied' or 'impotent' depended on whether they fell into one of five categories: children, the sick, the insane, 'defectives' and the 'aged and infirm'. [5] Michael Oliver contends that anyone who did not come under one or more of these headings was consequently classified as able-bodied; however Michael Rose has suggested that in practice all adult paupers between the ages of sixteen and seventy were automatically regarded as able-bodied unless they were permanently incapacitated in some way.[6] Outdoor relief for those in short-term need was not banned by the new legislation and indeed remained available to the Poor Law Commissioners, who replaced the previous Poor Law Boards. There was also staunch resistance to the new system, particularly in the industrial north and the midlands.[7] However, the Act was generally interpreted as applying to all claimants and so institutional relief in the form of workhouse residence was often the main or even only form of support available to paupers in many parts of the country.

Deaf people and the New Poor Law

Precisely how deaf people were treated under the Poor Law in any of its forms is unclear but they certainly gained no preferential treatment after 1834. Whether they were treated as 'deserving' or 'undeserving' poor is unclear and indeed their status is open to some debate. On the one hand, their deafness (particularly for those classified as 'deaf and dumb'), coupled with historical perceptions of deafness as a 'handicap' or impairment, would suggest they might have been regarded as impotent and therefore deserving. However, in practical terms, deafness is no barrier to performing any number of useful and productive jobs, so a more equal – but ultimately harsher – interpretation might have seen them classed as indolent and therefore undeserving. 'Infirmities' was one of three classifications included in Gilbert's Act of 1872 that identified someone as being 'deserving' and thus eligible to claim indoor relief via the workhouse (the others were old age and sickness). Thus it is quite possible that deafness was regarded as an infirmity because of the inability to hear. However, Gilbert's Act carried the caveat that such claimants should also be 'unable to acquire a maintenance by their labour' – in effect be incapable of work.[8] However, unless they suffered some other impairment, deaf people were not physically incapable of undertaking useful employment, and therefore might have been considered 'able-bodied'. Many deaf people were in effect 'able bodied' in terms of performing various types of manual work, no matter what difficulties may have existed in terms of communicating with hearing colleagues. However, many were unskilled or untrained, as there was little or no education or vocational training for the majority of deaf people at this time. Nevertheless, deafness in itself did not render deaf people 'unable to acquire a maintenance by their labour'. So how deaf people were treated under the more relaxed regime of the Old Poor Law is uncertain. However, their position was much clearer after 1834.

Lees identifies three categories of paupers who were able to enter the work-houses under the new system: the able-bodied; the aged and infirm; the insane, lunatics and idiots. Deaf people might have been categorised as 'able-bodied', through their ability to perform certain types of work, or as 'infirm', due to their deafness. Lees also notes that, somewhat perversely, all but the indolent and undeserving able-bodied were seen as 'unproductive defectives' after 1834, but this does not help to clarify the position of deaf paupers.[9] Where they seen able-bodied and therefore indolent, or where they classed as defective and thus 'unproductive'? In practical terms it is unlikely to have made much difference to their lives, as there was no obvious differentiation in the way all workhouse residents were treated and so these categorisations did not bring benefits to anyone. Deaf people (particularly those who could not speak – the 'deaf and dumb') thus found themselves in a disadvantageous position under the New Poor Law, whether they were regarded as 'deserving' or 'undeserving', with many deaf paupers subjected to the harsh realities of the life under the New Poor Law. Deaf historian Arthur Dimmock contends that many deaf people who could work were placed in the workhouse for no other reason than their deafness, and not because of any physical inability or unwillingness to work. Those who found themselves in the workhouses effectively became inno-cent victims of the wider changes in attitudes towards the poor and paupers, punished for their deafness rather than for being indolent.[10]

Precise figures on the number of deaf people who found themselves in this situation are not readily available and there is a vast amount of territory that remains unexplored concerning deaf people and the Poor Law. However there is clear evidence that deaf people found themselves in the workhouses. *The National Index of Paupers in Workhouses in 1861* offers a rare insight into the way deaf people were treated by the Poor Law Commissioners after 1834. Based on the 1861 Census, the *Index* contains information on all 14,200 adult paupers resident in English and Welsh workhouses at the time the census was taken. As well as giving names and the length of time each pauper had been resident in the workhouse, 'the reason assigned why the Pauper in each case is unable to maintain himself or herself' is also given. The use of 'unable to main-tain' has echoes of Knatchbull's Act and may suggest that all those recorded in the *Index* were considered to be 'deserving'; there are certainly no residents who are explicitly classified as 'indolent'. A 10 per cent sample of the *Index* reveals twenty-three workhouse inmates who were described as 'deaf and dumb'; a simple extrapolation would suggest at least 230 long-term deaf resi-dents in workhouses in 1861.[11] Only five of the sample had other physical or mental conditions which would prevent them from working. These included one who was blind, two with 'defective sight', one 'cripple' and one 'idiot'; in addition, one woman was listed as being 'deaf and dumb, and having an illegiti-mate child'. The remaining seventeen are merely described as 'deaf and dumb', suggesting they were capable of working. Examples of deaf people in work-houses were found from all parts of England, indicating some consistency in the way deaf people were being treated under the New Poor Law.

The extrapolation of 230 deaf residents in workhouses does not provide a particularly large sample from which to determine wider trends, such as vary-ing application of the Poor Law in different parts of the country, but the true figure was undoubtedly much higher. The figures cited from the *National Index of Paupers* relate only to adults (i.e. those over sixteen years of age) who had been resident in the workhouse for a period of five years or more. Therefore, it is virtually certain that there were a number of deaf people who were not recorded by this survey, including those who had been in the workhouses for less than five years or who were under sixteen years of age at the time of the 1861 Census. Indeed Raymond Lee suggests a much higher figure of around 1,300 deaf workhouse inmates at that time, based on an 1896 source which claimed that 6.7 per cent of a curiously precise total deaf population of 19,501 were residing in the workhouses in 1861.[12] Although these figures must be taken with some caution, it is undeniable that deaf people were being forced to enter workhouses and for no apparent reason other than their deafness. For those who are recorded, the length of time they had been receiving poor relief in the workhouse varied between seven and twenty-two years. Thomas Barlow, who had been in the workhouse in Stamford in Lincolnshire since 1839, was described as 'deaf, dumb and a cripple'. This suggests that his deafness was not necessarily the only factor in his inability to support himself. However, Mary Coram of Tavistock and Caroline Fox of Sheppey had both been receiving Poor Relief in their respective workhouses for sixteen years, and both were described simply as 'deaf and dumb'.

Although the age of workhouse inmates was not recorded, 'old' and 'aged' were regularly given as the reasons for individuals being admitted to the work-house. Some of those deaf persons listed in the *Index* may have been too old to work, but there is nothing to suggest this was the case. This evidence there-fore suggests that over a quarter of a century after the change in the Poor Law, deaf people were still being placed in workhouses solely on the basis of their deafness. This supports Dimmock's assertion that deaf people were being placed in the workhouse because of their deafness, rather than an inability to work. A second survey conducted in 1887 showed a remarkably similar situ-ation a quarter century later, with 1,289 paupers classed as 'deaf and dumb' resident in workhouses and a further 586 receiving outdoor relief.[13] However, it is unlikely this was the fate of all deaf people who were capable of working.

Given the currently accepted ratios for the incidence of deafness in the late twentieth century mentioned in the previous chapter (one person in every seven having some degree of deafness and one in 1,000 being profoundly deaf) the number of deaf workhouse residents claimed by Lee does have some credibility. Applying the same ratio to the 14,200 paupers identified in the 1861 Index would indicate a figure of around 2,000 deaf people in the workhouses. Nevertheless, despite the misgivings of Dimmock, the number of deaf people found in workhouses in the 1861 census still represented a small proportion of the overall deaf population, as Lee's later source confirms. There are two possible reasons why this figure is so low. Firstly, Anne Borsay has shown that by 1849, only 11 per cent of non-able-bodied adults were resident in the workhouses, with the remainder receiving outdoor relief; the 1887 statistics cited above show that deaf people were not excluded from this form of poor relief.[14] Secondly, it is also very possible that the deaf welfare organisations that had emerged in the first half of the nineteenth century had achieved some degree of success in finding gainful employment for deaf people. This was one of the main reasons these organisations were set up and it was from these bodies that deaf clubs were to eventually emerge.

The establishment of Deaf Societies and Welfare Organisations

The first organisations for the care and welfare of deaf people appeared in Scotland during the early part of the nineteenth century.[15] Grant shows that these societies were typically set up either by religious denominations or as independent philanthropic ventures by former pupils of the emerging deaf schools. As well as providing practical support for deaf people in their daily lives, they also provided a location for continuing the friendships and social life first experienced in the deaf schools.[16] The Church of England was the major provider and supporter of deaf people, which was in keeping with the long tradition of church groups taking responsibility for the education and welfare of deaf people.[17] The change in the Poor Law then gave an added impetus to the development of welfare societies generally, not merely those that provided for deaf people.

Lees notes the growth in institutions and asylums from 1760 onwards, with asylums founded for such socially unacceptable groups as prostitutes, urchins and illegitimate children, all of whom were deemed worthy of moral and physical redemption.[18] Asylums provided not only a refuge from the causes of distress, but they were also meant to act as a mechanism for transformation and improvement: 'once in sanitized settings, the socially deviant would supposedly absorb discipline, order and Christian morals via osmosis'.[19] Although

deaf people were not necessarily seen as 'socially deviant', the prevailing attitude was certainly that deaf people's inability to hear made them 'abnormal'.
It is perhaps no coincidence that when the first free deaf school in Britain
opened in 1792 in London, it was named the Bermondsey Asylum for the
Deaf and Dumb Children of the Poor, nor that it was founded by a Minister
of the Anglican Church.[20] Deaf people were held to be in need of help and the
Churches, especially the Church of England, saw the salvation of deaf people
as a part of their moral crusade. The Church's position was that as deaf people
could not pray or hear the word of God as proclaimed through the Bible, they
could not find absolution and eternal life. In addition, deaf people also needed
more practical help, such as being found employment to keep them from the
workhouses. Therefore, it was a Christian duty to support and provide for
deaf people, as was shown by the Church of England's close involvement in
the development of organised deaf welfare.[21] Lysons cites three main motivating factors in the establishment of voluntary welfare societies for deaf people:
evangelism, mutual aid and philanthropy, and these were all evident in the
early development of deaf societies.[22]

Although individual deaf societies began to emerge across Britain from the
1820s, the first organised network of deaf societies only appeared soon after
the change in the Poor Law and as a direct response to the suffering deaf people
were experiencing as a result. The Institution for providing Employment,
Relief and Religious Instruction for the Deaf and Dumb was founded in
London in 1841, later changing its title to The Royal Association in Aid of Deaf
People (RAD).[23] Formed as a charitable organisation, the Institution modelled
itself on the Edinburgh Deaf Society established in the mid 1820s and set up
missions across south-east England to provide training in various trades such
as printing, bookbinding and shoemaking. The Institution's declared intention was keeping deaf people out of the workhouses by providing a means
by which they could support themselves. Initially, only men were trained,
but later dressmaking and needlework was introduced for women. The initial
provision of training solely for men may have resulted from the stricter rules
for receiving assistance applied to males by the Poor Law Commissioners, thus
increasing the need to provide deaf men with an escape route from the stric-
tures of the workhouse.[24] Financial difficulties soon saw the vocational training
scheme suspended, despite its success in turning out well-trained craftsmen.
Many deaf people ended up back in the workhouses, and so efforts were made
to re-establish the missions. In 1854, the organisation re-emerged as The
Association in Aid of the Deaf and Dumb (AADD), this time with a much
more evangelical focus. The role of Missioners was introduced, to provide care
and welfare for the deaf people in their area through religious instruction and

education, although their role developed over time. Vocational training was no longer provided, although Missioners did try to find work and apprenticeships for deaf people. They also acted as advocates and advisors to deaf people in their areas, their most vital function being to provide interpreting between deaf and hearing people.

The influence of the Anglican Church in the work of the missions was evident from the start, as all those receiving support had to agree to attend regular church services and receive compulsory religious instruction. The AADD appointed their own deaf chaplain in 1851, and established a church solely for deaf people in London in 1890. Britain's first deaf church, St Saviour's, was built on Oxford Street, on a site now occupied by Selfridges department store. [25] Many other deaf societies followed suit in establishing missions, emphasising the religious basis and focus of much of the welfare provided for deaf people. Whilst the provision of church services and religious instruction was the primary purpose of many of the missions, they also served a social function. Informal gatherings began to occur as a natural extension of the regular religious meetings, and many missions began to arrange outings for their members. The Red Lion Square Deaf Mission in London was one example of the way such missions developed in places for social interaction. The original religious function of the Mission gradually became less important to its deaf users than the social role that resulted from bringing deaf people together, and this process of change was repeated in many other deaf missions. [26] Through the establishment of missions, and subsequently deaf clubs, deaf people were brought together, and consequently a sense of community based on shared interests, experience and communication methods began to be fostered. Taylor contends that the provision of a place for deaf people to meet and socialise was another important factor motivating those who set up the deaf societies from which deaf clubs emerged. [27] As missions for deaf people spread across the country, so the opportunities for community development through shared religious and leisure activities increased. Grant has identified at least thirty-six missions and deaf societies in existence across Britain by 1890, mostly in the cities and larger towns such as London, Birmingham, Liverpool and Manchester where there was a large deaf population. Others were set up in towns such as Doncaster that housed the major deaf schools. [28]

The work of the AADD was confined to London and the south east, but the services provided by the Institution were to become a major influence on the work of later organisations such as the British Deaf Association (BDA) and the Royal National Institute for Deaf People (RNID). Deaf societies emerged across the country during the late nineteenth and early twentieth centuries, mostly as independent organisations developed along similar lines to the

AADD model by churchmen and religious groups. The missions and societies operated under a range of titles, such as The Mission to the Deaf and Dumb of the Diocese of Carlisle, The Yorkshire Institution for the Adult Deaf and Dumb and The Salford and Manchester Deaf and Dumb Benevolent Association.[29] These voluntary societies provided varying degrees of welfare support for the local deaf population and appointed a superintendent to perform the same roles as the Missioners. Eventually, the title of Missioner came to be used for all those involved in such work, and as the premises from which they worked developed a social function, these became known as deaf clubs or Deaf Institutes. The Missioners often came from a religious background and were mostly but not exclusively hearing, and deaf people were often actively involved in delivering the services provided by the missions. The missions recognised the need for sign language as a means of communication between deaf and hearing people, and were promoters of its use. Sign language was recognised by many churchmen as being the most appropriate means of communication between deaf and hearing people, and it was used particularly in the missions' religious work. For example, the majority of missions included the provision of interpreted church services for their deaf congregations. By providing access to religious services through sign language, the Missioners were able to fulfil one of their principal functions – the spiritual salvation of deaf people. The various Christian churches have a long history of using forms of signed communication with deaf people, based on the organised sign systems used by several silent monastic orders. French clerics such as the Abbé de l'Épée and the Abbé Sicard were also instrumental in helping to formalise local versions of signed language into standard patterns of communication for educational purposes. In doing so, the churches played a major role in promoting sign language as the most appropriate form of communication for profoundly deaf people.[30]

The foundation of the British Deaf and Dumb Association (now the BDA) in 1890 was an important development in deaf welfare and subsequently deaf leisure, not least because the BDA was the first truly national organisation of deaf people with a deaf leadership.[31] In some respects, the establishment of a national – rather than local or regional – association for deaf people might be seen as a late development in relation to other disadvantaged groups. For example, the Royal National Institute for the Blind was established in 1868. However, in other respects, deaf organisations were either ahead of other groups or at least keeping pace. The National Society for the Prevention of Cruelty to Children was established in London in 1884, whilst the first ragged school for the poor of London was only founded by Barnardo in 1867 – over seventy years after a similar school was set up for deaf children. In another context, the deaf welfare organisations were no different to other welfare groups, as both the NSPCC and Barnardos were established by churchmen. The most important difference, though, was that the BDA was instigated by those who were to use its services, rather than by well-meaning outsiders. The driving force in the establishment of the BDA was Francis Maginn, a Missioner in Ireland who was himself deaf.[32] As the fledgling organisation developed in the early years of the twentieth century, they worked closely with the existing missions and deaf societies in which many of their members were found. The BDA looked to establish a branch in every city and major town, and the logical place to base their activities was in the network of local deaf societies and deaf clubs. As a result, most deaf clubs became affiliated to the BDA, with a club member serving as branch secretary and using the deaf club as the centre for his or her activities. This link to the BDA remained a feature of deaf club life throughout the twentieth century, with Grant citing the existence of 178 BDA branches based in deaf clubs in 1990.[33] Although the BDA was not usually formally involved in the running of deaf clubs, having a member acting as BDA branch secretary meant that the distinction between the activities of the deaf clubs and the BDA branches was often blurred. The branch secretary's responsibilities included collecting subscriptions, keeping the members informed of BDA activities, seeking the views of BDA members on important policy issues, and voting on behalf of the club's BDA members at the annual conference. As an illustration of the symbiotic nature of the BDA and deaf clubs, all BDA branches were required to raise money for the organisation as part of the latter's centenary celebrations in 1990.[34] This meant that many deaf clubs organised fundraising events for the BDA appeal as part of their normal schedule of activities. To all intents and purposes, the deaf club and the BDA branch were one and the same, with news of deaf club activities disseminated around the country through the pages of the BDA's newspaper, *British Deaf News*, with reports and information usually provided by the club's BDA branch secretary. The reports were even included in pages entitled 'Around the Clubs' rather than being presented as BDA branch reports.

Deaf clubs in north-west England

The latter part of this book focuses on a case study of deaf leisure in north-west England, and outlining the development of deaf clubs in the region will help to contextualise that analysis as well as serving as an example of wider national trends. As recently as 2003, there were twenty-eight active deaf clubs within the north west of England; that is clubs open to members at least one night per week.[35] Evidence drawn from *British Deaf News* (*BDN*) shows that virtually all of these clubs were in existence throughout the post-war period, and evidence from earlier deaf newspapers and periodicals shows that many of these clubs had been around for much longer. The clubs provided various leisure activities and facilities, and catered for deaf people of all ages, with many clubs having youth and pensioner sections. Drinking in the club bar and playing darts, snooker and bingo formed the regular staples of weekly deaf club activity throughout the post-war period. Deaf clubs also arranged a wide range of other leisure and sporting activities for members, both inside and outside the premises of the deaf club and these are discussed later in this book.

Manchester provides useful examples of the place of the missions and deaf societies within a wider expansion of welfare provision by voluntary charities, and the way in which deaf clubs developed as the social arms of missions for deaf people. Peter Shapely has shown that as many as 120 welfare organisations were founded in the city during the late eighteenth and early nineteenth centuries.[36] The Manchester Deaf and Dumb Institute was just one of a number of such organisations founded during this period, such as Henshaw's Blind Society, the Orphanage and Training School for Destitute Girls and the Discharged Prisoners Aid Society and a number of charitable hospitals and dispensaries appeared between 1795 and 1850. Alderman Chesters-Thompson was typical of the important and influential businessmen and philanthropists who supported voluntary welfare in the city during the second half of the nineteenth century. By 1891, Chesters-Thompson was 'a vice-president of Manchester Royal Infirmary, and one of the largest subscribers to the Manchester Eye Hospital, the Ancoats Dispensary and the Convalescent Home in Southport'.[37] He was also, amongst other philanthropic ventures, 'one of the chief supporters of the Adult Deaf and Dumb institution, of the Cotton Districts Convalescent Fund and the Day Nursery for the Children of Widows'.[38] Chesters-Thompson's decision to support deaf welfare in the city placed deaf people on an equal footing with other 'deserving unfortunates' and helped strengthen opinions that deaf people were worthy recipients of charity.

The Deaf Institute's formal charitable status was an important factor, as voluntary charities were not subject to the restraints applied by the 1819 Charitable Trusts Act.[39] This meant they and their supporters could employ a range of novel techniques to their fundraising activities, and as Shapely shows, providing entertainment in return for donations became an important aspect of their work. Dinners, Flag Days, concerts, bazaars and tea parties were amongst the activities used as devices to raise public awareness of the various charities and to attract donations, whilst providing donators with some amusement in return. Paying to take part in a balloon ascent was one of the innovatory ways in which people were encouraged to make donations in aid of Manchester Royal Infirmary. Manchester Oddfellows staged a public procession followed by a dinner to celebrate the opening of a new Deaf School in Old Trafford, Manchester in 1837. The Oddfellows had been involved in raising money to build the school, and they extended an invitation to 'any of their friends who wish to favour them' to join them in the celebratory dinner, on purchase of a ticket.[40] The development and support of welfare support for deaf people thus fitted well into the general philanthropic provision within the growing urban environment of Manchester. Even in their physical spaces, deaf organisations were linked to other deserving causes. When the new Deaf School opened in 1837, the site was shared with the new home of Henshaw's Society for the Blind, although the two organisations had separate but identical buildings.[41] However, this arrangement was to have financial implications for the Deaf School. The Blind Society was commonly known by the abbreviated title of 'Henshaws', and following the move to a shared site with the Deaf School, the two organisations came to be thought of as a single entity with a single title. The consequence for the Deaf School was that donations and bequests were regularly made to 'Henshaws', which meant that all such funds went to the Blind Society of that name, and money that may have been intended for the Deaf School, either for their sole use or to be shared with the Blind Society, was unintentionally misdirected.[42]

The first deaf society in Manchester was founded in 1846 by James Herriot, a deaf tailor from Edinburgh.[43] Herriot had been involved in setting up the deaf association in his home city, and he was keen to see a similar venture established in Manchester. His shop became a meeting point for local deaf people who came to Herriot for help and advice on a range of matters, and an *ad hoc* but unofficial Mission became established in the rooms above Herriot's shop. Here, deaf people came to meet and socialise with other deaf people, as well as seeking practical help in obtaining jobs and information. The informal deaf society was launched as an official organisation in 1849, under the title of the Manchester and Salford Adult Deaf and Dumb Benevolent Society and the first deaf centre was established in central Manchester the following year, as the Manchester Adult Deaf and Dumb Institute.[44]

Fundraising was one of the issues that saw Herriot's non-denominational organisation face opposition from the board of the Old Trafford Deaf School, which was run by the Church of England.[45] Herriot's fundraising was seen to be depriving the school of funds, and so an alternative, strictly denominational association was set up in 1854, as the Manchester Adult Deaf and Dumb Society.[46] The similarity between the titles of the two organisations was almost certainly not a coincidence, as the new body set out to portray themselves as the legitimate organisation for the welfare of the city's deaf population. Despite the efforts of the Old Trafford society and its Church of England based

backers, Herriot's group continued to grow and moved to more suitable premises in Quay Street, Manchester in the 1870s, where it remained for almost
one hundred years. No matter what the motives of those involved in setting up
deaf societies, a deaf club almost invariably emerged once deaf people began
to meet in the missions and societies. Whilst the work of the Old Trafford
society remained firmly based on religious instruction and spiritual care, a
social element also developed as a consequence of deaf people being brought
together. From its inception, Herriot's more secular group had provided social
as well as practical facilities and services for its members, and both the rival
societies came to establish dedicated social clubs for their members.

The main differences between the two organisations were those of religious
background, the membership of their controlling bodies and the support they
gave for what they perceived to be the most suitable method of education for
deaf children. Herriot's group was a loose cross-denominational gathering of
people from various Nonconformist backgrounds, whilst the Old Trafford
society was staunchly Church of England. The Church of England group
was run by an exclusively hearing Board and hearing staff, whilst although
Herriot's group had a mostly hearing management board, deaf people were
heavily involved in the running of their own organisation. Herriot was a firm
believer in the use of sign language in the education for deaf children, whilst
the Old Trafford school, from which the Anglican society developed, was
firmly oralist. In many ways, the two Manchester organisations reflected the
policies and perspectives of the two national organisations for deaf people,
which emerged during the late nineteenth and early twentieth centuries. The
British Deaf Association played a similar role to Herriot's group in terms of
being an organisation run for and by deaf people, which gave support to the
use of sign language. The Royal National Institute for Deaf People, on the other
hand, came to have many similarities with the work of the Old Trafford society,
by being an organisation run by hearing people and strongly in favour of oral
education and the medical model of deafness. The involvement of religious
groups in Manchester's deaf welfare provision was extended when a Catholic
Deaf Society was established in 1929, based at St. Joseph's Deaf Centre, which
still serves as the city's Catholic deaf club. St Joseph's main work was been more
concerned with spiritual welfare, but the Deaf Centre also provided an important social focal point for deaf Catholics in the city.[47]

Although the sometimes acrimonious nature of the early development of
deaf welfare services in Manchester was not typical of the region as a whole,
the manner in which deaf clubs emerged as the social bodies of these philanthropic and spiritual ventures most certainly was. The various towns bordering
Manchester, such as Rochdale, Oldham, Ashton-under-Lyne and Stockport, all

had their own deaf clubs, which developed out of the missions set up in these towns by various religious groups during the late nineteenth and early twentieth centuries. This pattern was repeated across the north west, with missions and deaf clubs to be found in towns such as Bolton, Preston, Liverpool and St Helens from the late nineteenth century. Therefore, it is clear that deaf clubs have been an important feature of deaf life across the north west of England for well over a century and a half and that their roots were firmly based in broader charitable provision for disadvantaged social groups. However, the north west is not unique, with similar patterns of deaf club development being found across the UK. Although the religious basis of these organisations remained an important part of their work, the deaf clubs and societies themselves gradually became less focused on spiritual matters. This was illustrated when Manchester's two deaf welfare groups finally joined together to form the non-denominational Manchester Deaf Society in the 1970s after over a century of separate provision for the city's deaf population.[48] The gradual separation of the spiritual and temporal aspects of welfare provision for deaf people is perhaps best illustrated by an investigation of the development of deaf welfare during the twentieth century, and particularly in the period since the Second World War.

The role of the Missioners in sustaining deaf clubs

One of the main responsibilities of the Missioner was to act on behalf of deaf people on a daily basis. Based at the local deaf society or club, the Missioner provided practical support in all aspects of the lives of deaf people. As Grant points out: '[The Missioners'] role and importance within the deaf community, particularly in the early days, are difficult to exaggerate. They were friend, social worker and spiritual adviser to the deaf community, and inevitably became champions of its causes'.[49] As such, the Missioners provided an important link between the deaf and hearing worlds, acting as interpreter, advocate and supporter for the deaf people under their care. The practical aspects of the Missioners' work were so important for deaf people that the BDA supported the introduction of a training and qualification programme for those wishing to work with deaf people. The Deaf Welfare Examination Board (DWEB) was established in 1928, and resulted in the introduction of Deaf Welfare Officers (DWOs) to work alongside the Missioners.[50] The DWEB course standardised the welfare support to deaf people through successful candidates achieving one of two qualifications. The Deaf Welfare Certificate course lasted two years and covered all aspects of the welfare provision to deaf people, as well as teaching sign language to candidates. This allowed DWOs to provide the vital service of interpreting for deaf people in their interactions with the hearing world. The Diploma course required a third year of study, consisting of religious training which allowed DWOs to conduct some minor religious services and act as lay readers. Upon qualification, the DWOs were employed in the missions and deaf societies. In effect, the DWOs took over the practical elements of deaf welfare work, leaving the Missioners to organise the spiritual care of deaf people. Taking on much of the advocacy and interpreting role of the Missioners, the DWOs enjoyed a similarly respected position amongst the local deaf community, and one of their most important functions remained finding employment for deaf people. This support continued until the role of the Deaf Welfare Officer was subsumed within the new post of Social Worker for Deaf People during the 1970s.[51]

As well as providing practical support for deaf people and advocating on their behalf, the Missioners and the Deaf Welfare Officers also helped in the development of what came to be recognised as the 'deaf community', by bringing and encouraging deaf people to share activities in the deaf club. Both the Missioner and the Deaf Welfare Officer were pivotal in introducing new members into the life of the deaf club. However, once the work of the DWOs was taken over by Social Services Departments, the change in roles also led to a change in the way Social Workers supported the life – indeed the existence – of the deaf club. The Social Workers responsible for deaf people were no longer based in the deaf clubs, and their central role in the social life of the deaf community diminished. One major difference between the two roles was that religious matters were no longer the concern of those primarily responsible for deaf welfare, and there was a clear separation of the formal care provider network and religious groups. Another consequence of this separation of roles was that the Deaf Welfare Officer's active promotion of deaf club membership to younger deaf people no longer formed part of the more detached remit of the Social Worker for Deaf People. When responsibility for introducing young people into the deaf club was not taken on by deaf members to the same extent, this important – indeed vital – route into the social life provided by deaf clubs largely disappeared. Dwindling numbers of members subsequently had an adverse effect on the way deaf clubs had traditionally helped to bind the deaf community together.

The role of the deaf club in maintaining the deaf community

When arguing for the existence of a deaf community, Padden lists the three common features of a community as the sharing of common goals, having a shared geographical location and the freedom to organise the social life of its members, as first proposed by Hillery.[52] The previous chapter showed how the first criterion could be applied to the deaf community, and it can be argued that deaf clubs met the second and third criteria by providing a geographical basis for the deaf community, in which the community organised and conducted its social and leisure activities. The issue of choice is an important one both in the context of leisure generally and as a motivating factor for deaf people to become involved in the activities of deaf clubs. Hill, in attempting to define leisure, differentiates between the lack of choice involved in working life and the exercise of choice during free time: 'Leisure ... represents freedom, time in which individuals can "be themselves", when they can reveal their authentic nature as autonomous human beings'.[53]

Although many deaf people were actively encouraged to go along to their local deaf club by the Missioners and Deaf Welfare Officers, no one was forced to become a member. Deaf people still had a choice about becoming – and more importantly remaining – members of their local deaf club, and this was a choice many exercised. This provision and promotion of deaf club membership by outsiders – in this case the Missioners and Deaf Welfare Officers – closely mirrors the paternalistic nature of many working class leisure organisations during the late nineteenth and early twentieth centuries. Formal bodies such as Mechanics Institutes were seen as centres in which individuals and the broader community had access to rewarding and improving social activities, and deaf clubs served a similar purpose. In addition, deaf clubs provided their members with benefits that were not available to them in any other setting. As Padden states, there were definite and important attractions motivating deaf people to join deaf clubs:

> Deaf people consider social activities an important way of maintaining contact with other Deaf people ... One reason is certainly that Deaf people enjoy the company of other like-minded Deaf people. They feel they gain support and trusting companionship from other deaf people who share the same cultural beliefs and attitudes. [54]

This support and companionship was gained in the deaf clubs, and these clubs can be regarded as the geographical centres for the deaf community in lieu of any centralised home environment. In exercising choice through joining a deaf club, members thus found the opportunity to 'reveal their authentic nature'.[55] It was through involvement with the network of deaf clubs and their associated social activities that many deaf people came to accept their deafness as an important and positive part of their identity.[56] Deaf clubs also provided opportunities to join in the cultural activities of the deaf community that were not available elsewhere. The majority of deaf schools were gradually closed during the post-war period, increasingly so following the introduction of integrated education alongside hearing children under the 1981 Education Act. The loss of this entry route into the deaf community made the deaf clubs an even more important setting for the maintenance of communal deaf life based on the use of sign language. It was in the deaf clubs that many deaf people first experienced what might be regarded as a normal life; that is one in which they did not form a misrepresented and misunderstood minority.[57] This normality was based on a shared experience of deafness, which has long been a central pillar in establishing and maintaining the cultural life of the deaf community. The use of sign language also played an important role in this discovery and maintenance of group and self-identity, by allowing its users to express themselves fully and in the most appropriate manner. [58] The deaf club effectively provided a place of refuge for deaf people where they could withdraw from the stresses of living in a hearing world: 'the function of the [deaf] social club is to allow members to interact in a relaxed setting where there is no pressure for spoken language use and comprehension and where sign language provides the common communication medium'.[59]

For many deaf people, whether deaf from birth or deafened later in life, their first experience of sign language and the deaf community only came after they joined a deaf club or deaf organisation. This discovery of a new identity as a deaf person was a life changing effect for many who had previously felt isolated or psychologically incomplete.[60] Harris has shown that for many deaf people who were new to the deaf community, the deaf club was a place where they could both learn and practise their sign language skills.[61] The acquisition of this linguistic ability was vital for both communication and acceptance by existing members. Once in the deaf community, as represented by membership of the deaf club, individuals were able live in a deaf world. Here, they were able to take part in activities that brought them enjoyment, and to meet with others with similar experiences and backgrounds. Sharing and passing on experiences to others has long been a central part of deaf cultural life; part of being immersed in deaf culture was the passing on of the rules, codes of behaviour and history of the deaf community to following generations. As Padden states: 'entering into Deaf culture and becoming Deaf means learning all the appropriate ways to behave like a Deaf person'. [62]

The only way of learning 'how to behave like a Deaf person' was through social contact with other deaf people. The social elements of deaf communal life were very important, as deaf people did not generally have the chance to meet other deaf people on a regular basis other than in the deaf clubs. The deaf community – as represented by the membership and social life of the deaf clubs – thus provided an opportunity for deaf people to share and reconfirm

their status as members of a culturally distinct community. In having an identifiable pattern of behaviour by which members were recognised and accepted
by others, the deaf community was no different to any other community group.
Members of all such community groups have to 'fit in' in order to be accepted.[63]
However, the unique attribute of deaf clubs was that they provided members
with access to their shared history and culture that was not available anywhere
else. The incidence of around 90 to 95 per cent of deaf children being born to
one or more hearing parents means that there is very little opportunity for the
vertical transmission of history and culture; that is history and culture passed
down from preceding generations within the family unit.[64] Quite simply, deaf
children were not normally born directly into the life of the deaf community. It
is for this reason that the deaf community has only ever comprised a minority
of deaf people; access has had to be sought or provided. For those who did find
access to the deaf community, the initial transmission of shared deaf history
and culture tended to occur horizontally, through contact with deaf peers. It
was only after this horizontal introduction to deaf history and culture that a
route to vertical transmission became possible, through access to older deaf
people who also acted as important role models.

Social class and the deaf clubs

Research by Wilmott and Young in the 1960s suggested that social clubs were
more likely to attract members from a middle-class background than from the
working class.[65] Hill contends that for the working class: '… it is the more informal ties of neighbourhood, family and work that provide the foundations for
communal life'.[66] This is not to suggest that social clubs were the sole preserve
of the middle classes; the large number of working mens' clubs and political
clubs across working-class areas of many towns and cities in the post-war years
showed that social clubs played an important role in the leisure activities of
working-class people. Walvin argues that institutions such as Working Men's
Clubs emerged to provide the working class with 'a recreational challenge to
the dominance of the pub', and provided alternative leisure activities to merely
spending time drinking.[67] However, working-class people did not generally
join as wide a range of social interest clubs as the middle class did.

The deaf clubs appear to have adopted a mainly working-class ethos in the
shared leisure activities of their members, suggesting that the majority of their
members came from working class backgrounds. This is not to claim that all
deaf people are from working class families, but those from middle- or upper-
class backgrounds historically did not tend to join deaf clubs. Oral schools
actively discouraged the use of sign language and by extension contact with

the deaf community, and sign language was only used by those perceived to be educational failures who could not acquire clear speech and good lip-reading skills. Middle- and upper-class families were generally better placed to ensure that their deaf children were able to communicate effectively – often through a privately funded oral education – and so find a place in the hearing world, which did not include joining a deaf club. The employment opportunities open to sign language users also influenced the social class structure of deaf clubs. Research has shown that the majority of profoundly deaf people throughout the twentieth century were predominantly employed in manual or semi-skilled jobs.[68] In the deaf clubs, they mixed with others of a similar economic background. Therefore, it should not be surprising that deaf clubs reflected a working class ethos in at least some of their activities.

In the last quarter of the twentieth century, employment prospects for deaf sign language users began to improve and a 'deaf middle class' began to emerge, as pathways and opportunities into a variety of traditionally middle-class professions emerged. This came about largely through deaf sign language users gaining positions of power in the deaf organisations, and through the increased career opportunities afforded by improved access to college and university courses for sign language users. Government schemes such as 'Access to Work', which provides physical and technological support for deaf people in the workplace, and anti-discriminatory employment legislation, meant that many deaf people were able to enter careers previously closed to them. In doing so, they adopted not only the career aspirations of the middle classes, but also some of the social mores that pertain to their higher social status. It might be assumed that improved career opportunities for deaf people resulted in the social background of deaf club members becoming more mixed, but this has generally not been the case. Indeed, the emergence of a deaf middle class has been cited as one of the primary causes for the decline of deaf clubs in the last quarter of the twentieth century, both in Britain and America.[69] Despite being seen – and often serving – as community leaders and positive role models, it is felt that the new professionals have eschewed the values and aspirations expressed through deaf club activities. The deaf middle class have been roundly criticised for not taking a more active role in the deaf clubs, and some deaf professionals are not deaf club members. This supports the assertion by deaf club members themselves that their clubs – and indeed the wider deaf community – have essentially been working-class in nature. However, there are some marked differences between the way deaf clubs have functioned within the deaf community and the roles played by working class institutions in the hearing world.

The informal ties outlined by Hill which bound working-class people together through shared work, family and neighbourhood do not apply to deaf people in the same way. Deaf people do not necessarily work with other deaf people; they do not live in the same neighbourhoods; nor do they usually come from deaf families. There was also a need for the majority of working-class deaf people to organise their social lives in a structured way, through regular attendance at deaf clubs, which did not correspond to the findings of Wilmott and Young. Organisations such as social clubs might be seen to provide an escape from the normal world of daily life into an abnormal world far removed from the stresses and drudgery of daily life. Whilst this escapism element was also true of deaf clubs, an argument can be made that this happened for very different reasons to the way non-deaf people joined together socially. For many deaf people, particularly sign language users, full participation in the sound-based world of the hearing majority was denied to them because of communication difficulties. Lack of effective communication meant that sign language users working alongside hearing people were socially isolated from their colleagues and so did not take part in leisure activities with them outside the workplace. Even within the home and family, many profoundly deaf people had little or no access to everyday communication and socialisation. In effect, what the hearing majority considered to be normal life represented an abnormal way of life for sign language users, as this was ultimately socially, emotionally and psychologically unfulfilling. It was only within the confines of the deaf club, where sign language was the dominant form of communication, that any sort of 'normal' life could be led.

As was shown earlier, the sociability and attendant psychological benefits that arose from being able to meet and communicate with others of a similar background were the main attractions of the deaf club. Wise argues that the concept of 'home' is closely linked to feelings of identity derived from certain territories and that 'home' does not necessarily mean the same as 'the home'. He equates home to a sense of identity and the expression of culture, and contends that the presence of 'significant others' can provide feelings of family and home that do not necessarily relate to 'the home'.[70] Deaf clubs provide a clear illustration of this argument. In many respects, the deaf club served as a surrogate home for profoundly deaf people, providing social and emotional ties that did not necessarily exist within the members' biological families. The deaf club took the place of the informal ties that were found in the hearing world. Instead, the clubs provided an opportunity to communicate and socialise that was missing in virtually all other aspects of a deaf sign language user's life. The deaf club not only provided its members with a refuge from the hearing world's version of the real world, but it also provided a socially more rewarding form of 'normality' for its members. In effect, being in the deaf club replaced the real world of daily life with an alternative 'deaf real world' that more closely reflected the experiences of daily socialisation hearing people took for granted. Therefore, social class was not as important as a criterion for membership as the ability and the desire to communicate in sign language and to meet with others from a similar background.

Deaf clubs were – in theory at least – historically open to all deaf people, regardless of gender, economic status or, in the post-war period, racial background. However, the membership of deaf clubs was almost exclusively white for most of the post-war period. It was only towards the last quarter of the twentieth century that some diversification in the ethnic background of members can be seen. Evidence of the involvement of deaf people from ethnic minority backgrounds is not given in the newspaper reports, but some insight can be gained from other factors. In photographs of club events or sports teams, no black or brown faces can be seen before the 1970s. Even then, these are very much a rarity. Nor do the reports include many names of participants that might suggest a non-British heritage. Whilst these sources are not completely reliable in this respect, they do indicate that people from ethnic minorities were no more likely to be found in deaf clubs than they were in other types of social clubs of the period. This is not to suggest that deaf clubs were overtly racist, but the racial constitution of their memberships is comparable to other social clubs catering for the wider community. Towards the end of the twentieth century, identifiable groups of non-white deaf people began to emerge across Britain. One example was the establishment of a deaf Asians social group in Manchester in 1995.[71] As society generally became more racially integrated towards the end of the twentieth century, the same process can be observed within deaf clubs, most obviously through the presence of Black and Asian members in photographs of sporting events.

The only type of acknowledged exclusivity practised by the deaf clubs seems to relate to the way clubs and societies were established on religious grounds.[72] This in itself may help to explain why members of ethnic minority groups do not appear to have joined deaf clubs, especially those deaf members of the immigrant families from the Indian sub-continent who moved en masse into the textile towns of northern England during the post-war period. It is only since the majority of deaf clubs lost their overt connections with religious groups that their membership has more obviously diversified on racial grounds. Membership may well have been restricted according to religious persuasion, but there was no other apparent means of selection used to determine who could become a member. When certain sections of the population were not found amongst deaf club members, this may have been due as much to their not choosing to join (for example deaf Muslims not wishing to join an overtly Anglican deaf club) as it was to their being refused membership. Why deaf people from ethnic backgrounds did not join deaf clubs is still open to debate but it is clear is that such deaf people were not generally found in deaf clubs throughout the majority of the post-war period. So the deaf community, as determined by membership of a deaf club, does not appear to be representative of the racial make-up of the broader population. In reality, the deaf community is too small to make any large scale selectivity practicable or desirable, and the role of the deaf club was to bring deaf people together, regardless of age, gender, class or even degree of deafness. Once inside the deaf club, members could then choose whom they wished to associate with, from the full range of members.

Deaf clubs were the focus of a wide range of social and leisure activities for their members, above and beyond the regular weekly club nights when members gathered together to socialise informally. As such, the clubs provided their members with ample opportunities to indulge in a variety of pastimes in the company of other deaf people with similar outlooks and life experiences. In doing so, deaf club members demonstrated the existence of a deaf community based on Hillery's three criteria outlined by Padden.[73] Members shared common goals, which derived from their shared experiences as deaf people and a desire to spend time with those of a similar background and outlook. These goals included sharing leisure activities, which took place both inside and outside the local deaf club. The deaf club therefore provided a geographical focus for these community activities, and these social activities were organised by the members themselves, not imposed by outsiders, thus allowing members to exercise control over this important aspect of their communal lives.

Although the development of deaf clubs can be traced back to a broader pattern of charitable provision for disadvantaged sections of society, they differed from other groups in that the deaf clubs helped to foster and actively promote notions of community and shared culture amongst their members. In this respect, deaf clubs came to have as much in common with working class structures such as Working Men's clubs as they did with the provision of welfare. However, the overall function of deaf clubs in sustaining the deaf community was no different from the role played by shared leisure and sport in all communities, as will be explored in the next chapter.

Notes

1   Borsay, A., *Disability and Social Policy in Britain since 1750* (Basingstoke: Palgrave, 2005); S. King, *Poverty and welfare in England: 1700–1850* (Manchester: Manchester University Press, 2000)

2   King, *Poverty and welfare*, pp. 21–25

3   Lees, L. H., *The solidarity of strangers: the English Poor Law and the people, 1700–1948* (Cambridge: Cambridge University Press, 1998), pp. 82–152

4   Gash, N., *The Age of Peel* (London: Edward Arnold, 1973)

5   Wright, D., 'Learning disability and the New Poor Law in England, 1834–1867' *Disability and Society* 15, 5 (2000), pp. 731–745

6   Oliver, *The politics of disablement*, p. 34; M. Rose, *The Relief of Poverty* (London: Macmillan, 1972), p. 14

7   King, *Poverty and welfare*, pp. 66–67

8   Borsay, *Disability and Social Policy*, p. 21

9   Lees, L. H., *The solidarity of strangers*, pp. 121–126

10   Dimmock, 'A brief history of the RAD', *Deaf History Journal*, Supplement X (2001) p. 16

11   The 10 per cent sample of the *National Index of Paupers in Workhouses in 1861* can be found on the UK and Ireland Genealogical Information Service website (http://www.genuki.org.uk/big/eng/Paupers)

12   Lee, R. (ed.), *A beginner's introduction to deaf history* (Feltham: British Deaf History Society, 2004), pp. 71–75

13   Lee, *Beginner's guide*, p. 71

14   Borsay, *Disability and Social Policy*, p. 25

15   Lysons, K. 'The development of local voluntary societies for adult deaf persons in England' in Gregory and Hartley, *Constructing deafness*, pp. 235–238

16   Grant, *Deaf advance*, pp. 1–13

17   McLoughlin, *A history of the education of the deaf*, provides a concise summary of the historical attitudes towards deafness and its effects, particularly amongst religious groups

18   Lees, *The solidarity of strangers*, p. 107

19   *Ibid.*, p. 107

20   Grant, *Deaf advance*, pp. 3–5; www.royalschoolfordeaf.kent.sch.uk/history.htm

21   McLoughlin, *The education of the deaf*

22   Lysons, 'The development of local voluntary societies', p. 236

23   Royal Association for Deaf People website: www.royaldeaf.org.uk; Dimmock, 'A brief history of the RAD', pp. 16–24

24   Lees, *The solidarity of strangers*, pp. 135–145

25   Dimmock, 'A brief history of the RAD', p. 18

26   O'Neill, R., 'Manchester and Salford Adult Deaf and Dumb Benevolent Society', *Deaf History Journal* (1997) Supplement II, pp. 24–25

27   Taylor, G., 'Deaf people, ethnic minorities and social policy' in Gregory and Hartley, *Constructing deafness*, p. 242

28   Grant, *Deaf advance*, p. 11

29   *Ibid.*, pp. 11–12

30   See D.C. Baynton, *Forbidden signs* (Chicago: University of Chicago Press, 1996); H. Lane, *When the mind hears* (London: Vantage, 1984)

31   Grant's *Deaf advance* is the official centenary history of the BDA, and provides extensive information on the foundation of the organisation

32   *Ibid.*, p. 5

33   *Ibid.*, p. 138

34   *British Deaf News (BDN)* 1990, January, p. 1

35   Royal Association for Deaf People website (www.royaldeaf.org.uk/ukclubs.htm)

36   Shapely, P., *Charity and power in Victorian Manchester* (Manchester: The Cheetham Society, 2000), pp. 141–143

37   *Ibid.*, p. 103

38   *Ibid.*, p. 103

39   *Ibid.*, pp. 23–24

40   *Ibid.*, pp. 30–32

41   Royal Deaf School, Manchester: www.rsdmanchester.org/history

42   Woolley, D., *Manchester memoirs: a pictorial record of the Manchester School for the Deaf* (Doncaster: British Deaf History Society, 2001), pp. 1–2

43   O'Neill, 'Manchester and Salford Society', pp. 15–31

44   Shapely, *Charity and power*, p. 23

45   O'Neill, 'Manchester and Salford Society', pp. 24–25

46   For simplicity, 'The Manchester and Salford Adult Deaf and Dumb Benevolent Society' is referred to as 'Herriot's group', whilst the 'The Old Trafford society' is used for 'The Manchester Adult Deaf and Dumb Society'

47   Catholic Deaf Association website: www.cda-uk.com

48   *British Deaf News* 1975, pp. 88, 158, 189

49   Grant, *Deaf advance*, p. 6

50   Simpson, T.S., 'A stimulus to learning, a measure of ability' in Gregory and Hartley, *Constructing deafness*, pp. 217–225

51   Grant, *Deaf advance*, pp. 58–59

52   Padden, 'The deaf community and the culture of deaf people', p. 3

53   Hill, *Sport, leisure and culture*, p. 6

54   Padden, 'The deaf community and the culture of deaf people', p. 10

55   Hill, *Sport, leisure and culture*, p. 6

56   Ladd, 'The modern deaf community'; Mason, 'School experiences'

57   Brien, D., 'Is there a deaf culture?' in Gregory and Hartley, *Constructing deafness*, p. 50

58   Harris, *The cultural meaning of deafness*

59   Kyle and Woll, *Sign language*, p. 11

60   For example, see Mason, 'School experiences'; M. Woolley, 'Signs of strife'

61   Harris, *The cultural meaning of deafness*, p. 126

62   Padden, 'The deaf community and the culture of deaf people', p. 44

63   Bourke, J., *Working class cultures in Britain 1890–1960* (London: Routledge, 1994) and Anderson, *Imagined communities*

64   Lane *et al.*, *A journey into the DEAF-WORLD*, p. 30

65   Wilmott, P. and M. Young, *Family and kinship in a London suburb* (London: Routledge and Kegan Paul, 1960)

66   Hill, *Sport, Leisure and culture*, p. 132

67   Walvin, J., *Leisure and society, 1830–1950* (London: Longman, 1978), p. 41

68   Young *et al.*, *Looking on*; G. Montgomery and K. Laidlaw, *Occupational Dissonance and discrimination in the employment of deaf people* (Edinburgh: Scottish Workshop Publications, 1993)

69   Padden, C., 'From the cultural to the bi-cultural: the modern deaf community' in I. Parasnis (ed.), *Cultural and language diversity and the deaf experience* (Cambridge: Cambridge University Press 1996), pp. 84–85

70   Wise, 'Home: territory and identity'

71   *BDN* 1995, September, p. 23

72   There has also been a Jewish Deaf Club in London for a number of years

73   Padden, 'The deaf community and the culture of deaf people', p. 3

4

SUSTAINING COMMUNITIES THROUGH SHARED LEISURE AND SPORT

It is clear that deaf clubs played a central role in helping to sustain and rein-force notions of identity amongst deaf people. This was of particular impor-tance in helping to establish and recognise deaf sign language users as members of a distinct social, cultural and linguistic community. The way in which this expression of culture and identity manifested itself and was shared more widely through the pages of *British Deaf News* will be described in detail in subsequent chapters. At this stage, it is important to investigate how shared leisure and sport can help to maintain communities, and to relate these concepts to the activities of the deaf community.

As has already been established, communities can be established through a number of shared factors, such as social, geographic, relational and political connections.[1] Feelings of community may result from shared residence or alter-natively through shared characteristics; both elements need not be shared in order to form a community. A sense of community identity can develop simply by living in a particular area, without members of the community necessar-ily sharing characteristics with their neighbours.[2] On the other hand, shared residence does not lead to a sense of community unless the residents also share some form of common identity. As Meegan and Mitchell point out, there can often be a very real distinction between sharing a common neighbourhood and sharing a sense of community.[3] Lee and Newby argue that community can be based solely on shared identity – what they term 'communion'.[4] In this model, a sense of community can be derived within a 'local social system', in which individuals are linked by social networks.[5] Two examples of local social systems from the deaf world were the residential deaf schools and the deaf clubs, both of which provided deaf people with access to social networks. It was through attendance at a deaf school that the majority of deaf people first came to develop feelings of shared identity and found access to the wider deaf community. As the history of deaf club development has illustrated, a major motivations for joining a deaf club was to maintain the social bonds that deaf people developed whilst attending a deaf school. Once school days were over, unless they joined a local deaf club, deaf people returned to a world in which they were mostly isolated from each other.

Choosing to join a deaf club provided another way to access this community of like-minded individuals, even if no bonds with former pupils were involved. The deaf clubs thus served as a means of maintaining and continuing existing connections with the deaf community, as well as acting as a catalyst for the formation of that community. As was shown in the previous chapter, deaf people identified with each other through the shared characteristics of their deafness rather than because of where they lived. So deaf clubs provided both a geographical centre for the deaf community and a social network through which existing notions of community and identity could be maintained.

A shared interest in various leisure pursuits is one of the most common characteristics that can contribute to the formation of a community. In this type of 'interest community', it is not necessary to live close to other members for as Crow and Allen point out, 'interest communities may be geographically dispersed'.[6] The sense of 'communion' that is shared through the social aspects of these types of community is often an essential factor in the formation and maintenance of the community and provides access to the networks posited by Lee and Newby. Once inside such a network, communication with other members is vital if a sense of shared identity and interests is to be developed and sustained. This is one of the reasons why so many types of interest communities not only communicate face to face but through newsletters, magazines and other forms of publication. For those deaf people who are unable to communicate effectively with the hearing population, contact with other deaf people is vital for reinforcing notions of community membership. The social life provided by the deaf clubs, based as it was on sign language use, provided a means of access to others who shared the same medium of communication and thus had similar experiences, perspectives and expectations.[7]

Given the social basis of many forms of community, it is apparent that each community will have its own patterns of behaviour and social mores, by which members are defined and accepted. These might be regarded as the way each community expresses its own particular culture and the common identity of its members. Within this cultural identity, forms of leisure and recreation perform a central role: 'Sports and recreational activities [i.e. leisure] have formed a basic part of all cultures, including all racial groups and historical ages, because they are as fundamental a form of human expression as music, poetry and painting.'[8] It is those specific aspects of cultural behaviour directly related to leisure and sport that are of interest here, whilst acknowledging that there are many more forms of cultural expression.

Defining 'leisure'

Before discussing the role of leisure in building communities, it is necessary to construct a definition for 'leisure' to explain the way the term is understood within this book. Leisure can cover a broad range of activities from the sedentary at one end of the scale (for example reading, watching television or knitting) to the very energetic or dangerous (such as marathon running, mountain climbing or extreme sports) at the other.[9] In the interests of simplicity, a definition of leisure is used which recognises the diversity of activities the term may cover whilst focusing on those which involve some degree of socialisation. Therefore, leisure is taken to mean those recreation activities members of a community choose to take part in during their free time, either with other community members or as individuals, and which are seen to express or maintain the group's collective identity in some way. In the case of individuals, it is those activities in which they were identified as members of a specific community that will be considered. This is particularly relevant when investigating deaf people involved in leisure and sporting activities with hearing people. As will be shown later, in such circumstances the deafness of participants was often highlighted (and thus the individual's or group's identity established) even when this had no obvious relevance to the event being reported. Sport is just one element within a broader spectrum of leisure activity, and most of the factors relating to sport therefore apply more broadly to leisure. Those elements that relate more specifically to sport (for example, competition) will be dealt with later in this chapter. Leisure and sport provide a variety of forms of recreation, an important element of which is the attendant social life of all leisure and sport activities. Through this socialisation, group and self-identity can be found and reinforced, and a sense of communal attachment results.

The common factors put forward by Padden, Higgins and others when defining membership of the deaf community were shared experiences, shared identity and cultural expression.[10] The only places deaf people could be sure of encountering these three elements in the company of other deaf people were the deaf schools and the deaf clubs, and it was through these that membership of the deaf community was obtained. The rationale of deaf clubs was to provide their members with an opportunity to socialise with other deaf people, and so all the social activities of the clubs and their members can be regarded as leisure activities. In turn, these leisure activities played a central role in the development and maintenance of deaf communal life and in providing group and self-identity for their members. This book focuses on those aspects of deaf club life that were reported in *British Deaf News*, whilst acknowledging that these were not the sole constituents of deaf people's leisure pursuits. The more mundane and commonplace elements of the deaf clubs, such as playing bingo or members merely meeting to drink and chat, were equally important, but were not culturally distinct or unique to the deaf community. Instead, it was the types of activity that the deaf community chose to organise for itself that best illustrate cultural values and preferences and so it is these that will be investigated.

Many leisure and sport activities require the involvement of others (for example team sports or those activities which include some degree of competitiveness), whilst others can be pursued on an individual basis. However, even for the most solitary of leisure activities, participants still choose to come together in clubs and societies. Bishop and Hoggett put forward the following reasons to explain why participants gather together to share their interests: leisure 'provides a vehicle through which social exchange can take place'; groups provide opportunities to create collective products; groups provide opportunities for making friends and meeting people.[11] Even in those leisure activities that are essentially solitary pursuits (such as wine making, drawing or painting and gardening), socialisation with those who share one's interests provides important psychological and emotional rewards. Bishop and Hoggett illustrate how sharing interests can be regarded as 'communal leisure', which they define as 'collectives which are self-organized, productive and which, by and large, consume their own products'.[12] This definition can be seen to apply to deaf clubs. Members organised events on behalf of the deaf club, which they and other members then took part in collectively. The fourth key element identified by Bishop and Hoggett is mutual aid, examples of which can also be found in the history of the deaf clubs. These include social events held specifically to raise funds for free holidays for children and elderly members, decorating club rooms or the purchase of new equipment. This shared activity represents Crow and Allen's concept of an 'interest community' and the social elements provide the basis for 'communion' put forward by Lee and Newby as a means of gaining a shared identity.[13] It is not claimed here that taking part in leisure and sporting activities with other deaf people was the sole basis on which the deaf community exists. However, the exploration of deaf club activities in later chapters will show that these activities did play an important part in helping to foster and maintain a sense of communion between and amongst deaf club members. Whilst the deaf community itself is not merely an interest community, there are specific interest communities to be found within its range of social activities. Not all deaf people liked to take part in the same activities, or even with each other; however particular interest groups within the wider deaf community did help bring deaf people together from different geographical areas. This in turn helped to foster feelings of belonging to a greater body of people bonded together by more than a shared interest in a particular pastime or sport. With group identity comes a distinct way of behaving within the group or community, in order to fit in and be accepted. Rose and Kiger argue that 'identification with a group ... influence[s] an individual's social identity'.[14] Shared leisure allows for the transmission of values to participants, provides an entry route into specific groups and communities, and the leisure practices of the group integrate members into the society of the community. In Bourdieu's view, what he termed 'embodied actions' (a range of social practices such as engagement in leisure and sport with others) are 'the key to developing specific feelings which enable the individuals to be at ease with their self and with others of the same community'.[15] Thus, leisure and sport can assist individuals to develop a sense of both group and self-identity by providing access to an existing community of like-minded others.

An analysis of leisure and sport shows ways in which both internal and external factors impact on community development, based on ideas of 'sameness' and 'difference'. Rose and Kiger contend that 'groups form on the basis of difference' – that is, through being different to everyone who is not a member of the group.[16] The 'difference' of deaf people has historically been viewed in negative terms; their deafness has been regarded as a loss or impairment. However, the deaf community prefers to celebrate this difference, as illustrated by the debates concerning the place of hearing people within the deaf community.[17] Because hearing people do not share this difference, many commentators feel they cannot fully belong within the deaf community, no matter how positive their attitudes towards deafness and deaf people may be. Notions of difference can be reinforced internally through community members' choice of which leisure activities are enjoyed and with whom. Shogan shows how the 'partitioning' of leisure can constrain participants to those who are identified as belonging to a particular group or community. This partitioning can exclude those who are not deemed to belong to the group as a whole, but can also be used to differentiate within the group or community itself, for example on the basis of gender or skill and ability levels. Those who are not considered part of the 'in crowd' (on whatever basis) are not allowed to take part in the group's leisure activities.[18] It was in leisure settings that the criteria for membership of the deaf community found practical application. Unless an individual was accepted as a member of a deaf club, then such a person had no means of sharing in the leisure activities of the deaf community. Membership could be granted on a temporary basis (for example by invitation to a specific event) or was not necessarily dependent on deafness.

As several commentators have noted, hearing people have regularly been accepted into the deaf community although there is some difference of opinion on how deeply they are accepted. The important consideration was not necessarily deafness but was often one of acceptance; without this acceptance into the community, the active participation of apparent outsiders in the social life of the deaf clubs was impossible. Partitioning of leisure and sport can also take the form of self-advocacy or self-determination, with group members exercising power through their choices of activity on both individual and group levels.[19] As such, choice serves as an implicit political activity, in which a group hierarchy is established. This occurs through such factors as who decides what community members do; whom they share the activity with; where the activity takes place; and how the costs are met. In deaf clubs, responsibility for organising the social calendar was normally delegated to a committee comprised of club members, thus allowing the members themselves to exercise a degree of freedom and choice in their own activities.[20] As Padden and Humphries note, sport has been one of the few areas of deaf life in which deaf people have been able to exercise any control over all aspects of their involvement, and has served as a model of empowerment for deaf people.[21] To a large extent, the same has been true of the leisure activities organised by the deaf clubs. It may be more than coincidental that many of the deaf people who are currently leaders of the British deaf community have at one time or other closely involved in the organisation of deaf clubs and deaf sport.[22]

A sense of community can also be constructed through external influences, such as interaction with other communities. The most common expression of this is in competitive engagement with external groups, with the most obvious example being sporting events. In such contests, one community, as represented by a team or individual, is under symbolic attack from a group of 'outsiders'; Desmond Morris terms this aspect of sporting contests as 'stylized battle', in which sport serves as an alternative to war or conflict.[23] Alan Metcalfe provides an example of this process in a sporting context through his investigation of miners in the villages of north-east England. Despite having a strong internal sense of belonging to a community of which they were proud, the miners also needed to express their difference to others; sport provided a rare opportunity to do so.

'... sport was one of the few visible symbols that provided the miners with a positive view of themselves and with mechanisms for judging themselves against each other and the outside world'.[24] In such settings, it is not merely notions of community that become important, but also the way in which the community conducts itself; in other words, how the community expresses its cultural difference. It is through these contests that each group both gains and expresses their communal and cultural 'otherness' from non-members.[25] Communities and groups can also identify themselves via other competitive settings, for example by taking part in musical contests and Best Kept Village competitions. Whether sporting or not, all such contests pit the 'in crowd' as represented by a community against outsiders with whom they may share a common interest but not a common identity. Engagement with outsiders – that is, non-deaf groups and individuals – has been a regular feature of deaf leisure and sport, as will be outlined in more detail in chapters six and eight. In such events, the community identity of deaf participants was often strengthened because of the feelings of conflict that can be an inherent factor of deaf interaction with hearing people.[26] As Padden notes 'the existence of conflict brings out those aspects of the culture of deaf people that are unique and separate from other cultural groups', through which they emphasise the differences between themselves and their non-deaf counterparts.[27]

At this point, it is appropriate to mention briefly Bourdieu's concept of social capital and the role this plays in community bonding. While it is not the intention to revisit the many and various examples academics have put for forward to show how social capital can be acquired, the concept will be touched upon here and addressed again in later chapters to support the arguments relating to the specific example of communal deaf life. Bourdieu's basic premise – that a variety of benefits that he describes as four types of 'capital' are drawn from contact with others – can be seen to apply to the whole range of leisure activities of the deaf clubs.[28] Bourdieu includes amongst these benefits, both social capital and cultural capital, the acquisition and expression of which have been shown to play important roles in community development and maintenance.[29] Social capital is not an end in itself, merely a theoretical construction of what takes place naturally as communities form and develop. Shared leisure activities provide an ideal way of acquiring both social and cultural capital, with benefits drawn directly from involvement in social networks and group membership. Leisure offers the opportunity to gain both 'bonding' capital – that is with members of one's own community – and 'bridging' capital through engagement with other individuals and communities. In the context of the deaf community, bonding capital was gained through the activities of the deaf clubs. Deaf people were brought together locally, and members of different deaf clubs regularly met, with both types of engagement reinforcing notions of belonging to a larger community, whether regional, national or international. Bridging capital on the other hand could be the product of positive interaction with groups of hearing people, whether this took place on a formal or informal basis, and acted as a counterbalance to those instances that involved a degree of conflict or competition. One aspect of social capital acquisition that was often missing from the lives of deaf people was that found through the workplace. As was mentioned in the previous chapter, those deaf people who communicated via sign language had little or no access to the informal social interaction that forms an integral part of working life.[30] The lack of contact and communication between deaf and hearing colleagues meant that they did not join in shared social activities outside the workplace, and so bridging and bonding capital were not found through employment. Instead, sign language users joined deaf clubs and gained these through contact with other deaf people instead.

In addition, cultural capital was derived through the expression of cultural identifiers and the celebration of group identity that leisure and sport both bring.[31] Puttnam has described extensively the effects that a loss of social capital can have on the structure and continued existence of communities and this is of particular significance to the deaf community.[32] Puttnam argues that once social networks begin to erode (for whatever reason), then access to shared social capital is gradually lost and replaced by the predominance of solitary activities rather than those involving communal engagement. As social systems fail, 'communion' as espoused by Lee and Newby is lost and communal leisure no longer acts as a bonding mechanism within communities, on a variety of levels.[33] The ultimate consequence, in the opinion of Puttnam, is the decline of society in much broader terms. Evidence will be presented later to suggest that this process is already affecting deaf clubs and consequently diminishing their role within the deaf community. As the social networks of the deaf community have changed during the last quarter of the twentieth century and into the twenty-first, so the ways in which deaf people come together as a community have become increasingly diverse and fragmented. The effects of changes in deaf social life on the traditional concept of the deaf community will be discussed in the concluding section of this book.

As with many other aspects of shared leisure, sport plays an important part in building, developing and maintaining community bonds. As such, sport serves as a useful example of the social benefits that are an essential part of all leisure activities involving engagement with other people. Holt argues that sport is a means of maintaining and strengthening existing social ties, as well as providing an opportunity for attracting others of a similar background into the social circle of the group or community.[34] Sport is not merely about competition against outsiders; it also acts as a means of bonding those involved in or with a team. Sport does not merely 'reveal' underlying social values; it is a major mode of their expression. Sport is not a 'reflection' of some postulated essence of society, but is an integral part of society.[35] Sport can therefore be a powerful tool for preserving and maintaining the cultural life of a community, by acting as 'a source of cultural continuity between generations'.[36] The main motivations for participation in sport – sociability, emotional rewards, and group and self-identity – reflect the social basis of all sports. Indeed, sporting activity would be less attractive as a pastime without the social aspects of sports club membership. In all types and levels of sporting activity, pre- and post-match discussions are important elements in choosing which activity to take part in and with whom. Wohl and Pudelkiewicz contend that the most successful sporting organisations are those which best satisfy local needs for socialisation.[37] Bishop and Hoggett agree with this argument: 'even the most competitive sports clubs will tend to have a highly developed social side to the club's activity.'[38]

In this aspect, leisure and sport might be seen to function as a cultural subsystem of wider society.[39] Durkheim argued that increasing industrialisation and urbanisation in the developed world from the nineteenth century onwards resulted in a sense of social dislocation amongst many levels of society.[40] Modern leisure practices arose as an antidote to these upheavals to notions of shared community and identity as existing forms of life and work were replaced by more regimented lifestyles. Leisure – and increasingly during the nineteenth and early twentieth centuries, sport – assumed an important role in replacing former means of finding and celebrating communal identity that became subsumed within urbanised society.[41] As professional sport in particular became ever more popular throughout the twentieth century, attachment to sporting associations as a process for gaining a sense of belonging and community developed and expanded. Shared leisure and sport thus helps to mitigate, at a variety of local, regional and national levels, against the decline in society which Puttnam argues results from a loss of social capital.[42] Whilst society generally may decline and various means of acquiring social capital are lost as a result, leisure and sport remain an essential part of society and community. Membership of a social or sports club provides group identity both internally and externally, and strengthens notions of belonging to an interest community. Leisure celebrates sameness both within the community group and with outsiders; all participants share the same interests but are not in direct competition with each other, either as individuals or groups. Sport on the other hand celebrates sameness within the group (the team) but emphasises the group's difference through competition against outsiders.

Sport, as one facet of communal leisure activity, satisfies the need for identity reinforcement that Weiss argues is demonstrated by all human beings on a number of different levels.[43] Through the satisfaction of this need, the participant is able to find and maintain notions of identity on personal, internal and external levels. As Weiss concludes, such self-identification through interaction with others is a 'fundamental endeavour' of human behaviour and results in heightened self-esteem and confidence.[44] However, it is necessary for this identification to be confirmed and recognised, both by the participant and by others. Weiss identifies five types of recognition, which he classifies as 'social subjectivity':

1. as a member of a group (for example as a member of a team and therefore an 'insider')
2. in an assigned role (through the performance of a particular role at the request of other group members)
3. in an acquired role (through the acceptance of responsibility or the possession of a particular skill)
4. in a public role (by performing these roles in a public sphere on behalf of the group)
5. through personal identity (by being recognised as oneself within the group and not just as a member of a collective whole)

The sense of identity and derived benefits that results from such recognition is strengthened by the number of these roles an individual is associated with. A sense of self-identification and recognition can be also derived from a range of non-sporting leisure pursuits, which offer similar means of identification through formalised roles such as Chair, Treasurer or Secretary.

To illustrate how these types of recognition might be achieved in a sporting context, the example of a deaf footballer (referred to as 'Ben' for reasons of confidentiality) shows how he was able to derive a wide range of benefits through the status he gained as a deaf footballer. Despite retiring from football many years ago, he continues to enjoy an enhanced profile within the deaf community and he has a strong, positive self-identity as a deaf person.

1. as a member of a group – Ben was identified through his position as a member of the deaf club's football team
2. in an assigned role – he was the club's Treasurer and team captain
3. in an acquired role – he was the team's leading goal scorer and generally regarded as their best player, and as such his involvement was seen as vital to the team's success. He was also a member of the Great Britain deaf international team for several years
4. in a public role – he was invited for trials at his local professional football club despite being profoundly deaf, and was the subject of a newspaper feature as a result. This was a matter of pride amongst his local deaf community and was more widely reported through *British Deaf News*
5. through personal identity – he was regarded as a successful deaf person for a number of reasons, not merely because of his footballing achievements[45]

As he himself says 'I think that it [being a successful footballer] made me more confident. Maybe if I hadn't got involved with the football, I wouldn't be the person I am today'. [46]

Communal identity can often arise from attachment to a particular place, which the American geographer Yi-Fu Tuan christened 'topophilia' or the 'affective bond between people and place or setting'.[47] Tuan describes how such ties can develop for a variety of psychological reasons, but these can also come through engagement in the activities that take place in a particular setting, not merely the place itself. [48] Eyles contends that such attachments contribute to an enhanced quality of life, indicating the importance of topophilia in social and personal life.[49] John Bale examined the subject of topophilia in relation to football stadia, and found that the grounds of football clubs came to represent an alternative form of 'home' for many fans. Bale found that fans identify 'their club' as closely with the ground as they do with the team, and that the two cannot be separated. For those fans who develop an attachment to a particular stadium, they come to view the home ground as part of their heritage. When clubs are removed from their 'homes', then fans often feel a sense of dislocation and loss of identity.[50] The deaf clubs can be considered to serve a similar purpose within the deaf community, albeit that the priority is reversed; the deaf club represents firstly a place but also the body of people who attend that place and take part in its activities.

Topophilia can also arise from the events experienced and organised through a specific venue, not merely those activities that take place within a particular setting. Attachment to a particular place is thus extended beyond the mere physical space to include activities that are shared by group members away from the place itself. In terms of the deaf clubs, although the members may have had an attachment to the club's geographical location, the number of events that were arranged away from the club's premises suggests that a greater attachment was to the club as represented by a body of people. Members' sense of shared identity was derived as much from their participation in the club's social events, in the company of each other, as it was from attendance at the geographical location of the club. This issue will be discussed in more detail later in this book, when Montgomery Wise's contention that notions of 'home' and feeling 'at home' do not necessarily apply to the same physical space will be considered in relation to the concept of the deaf club.[51]

The role of leisure and sport in the deaf community

Within the deaf community, participation in leisure and sporting activities has served essentially the same purposes as it does in any other community.

Deaf people have taken part in leisure activities for the same reasons as anyone who is not deaf, and their deafness has been neither a demotivating nor a disabling factor: 'Their bodies are the same. Their minds are the same. Their desire to achieve and excel is the same.'[52] Deaf clubs provided their members with opportunities for recreation and socialisation that they could share with others of a similar background and interests. The importance of these shared leisure opportunities is emphasised by the lack of similar forms of relaxation in the daily lives of many deaf people. Geographical isolation from other sign language users and a lack of effective communication with the surrounding hearing majority meant that for many deaf club members, the social inter-course of everyday life was absent. The social aspects of deaf leisure and sport have always been an important motivating factor for those involved, and the deaf clubs were the main – or even sole – means by which a rewarding social life could be found.

Durkheim's principles for the development of leisure practices to counteract social dislocation can be seen to apply to deaf people and also arose as a direct result of increased urbanisation during the nineteenth and twentieth centuries.

As deaf people gathered together in towns and cities, schools and other institutions came into existence, which allowed deaf people to make contact with others of a similar background and to develop cultural attachments, such as a shared language. The reality of the deaf community as it is understood today developed as a direct consequence of deaf people being brought together in the schools and other welfare institutions. Once school days were over, deaf people looked for ways of continuing their social ties with each other and from this desire, deaf clubs were established. Whilst the majority of deaf people remained isolated within the hearing majority in their daily lives, deaf clubs were a direct response to this isolation, providing opportunities for socialising and sharing leisure activities that had not previously been available. As the later analyses of deaf people's leisure and sport will show, the concept of topophilia can be applied to deaf clubs. Members formed deep attachments not only to the deaf club as a physical space, but these feelings also extended to the activi-ties organised by the deaf clubs and to the people who took part in these activi-ties. Deaf club members gained an enhanced quality of life as a direct result of being members, and deaf clubs played an important – indeed vital – part in providing their members with a shared sense of identity that came through the activities they took part in together.

In terms of what deaf club members actually did together, the analyses of deaf club based leisure and sport illustrate that deaf people were no different to their hearing neighbours. They took part in similar social activities, indicat-ing that deaf people shared the same motivations for choosing various leisure and sporting events and derived similar benefits from doing so. Without the existence of deaf clubs and the access to leisure activities they provided, it is difficult to see how else the physical and emotional needs provided by the recreational and social aspects of leisure could have been met as effectively. As will be shown, sport has been a major element of deaf leisure and it is here that some differences with other groups can be noted. Stewart highlights the way in which deaf sport provides an alternative view of deafness to the dominant deficit model which only sees deafness in terms of loss: 'deaf sport emphasises the honour of being deaf, whereas society tends to focus on the adversity of deafness'.[53] The same could be claimed for other deaf club activities, as only those who were accepted into the clubs were allowed to take part. Other benefits derived from deaf sport included the element of choice, which was not always a factor in other aspects of deaf people's daily lives. Choice could be expressed through deciding which sports to take part in, and with whom, whilst self-determination came through involvement in the organisation and control of deaf sporting bodies.[54] Participation in deaf leisure and sport also provided deaf people with the means to be recognised as deaf community members, on the basis described by Weiss.[55] The social benefits derived within the community matched those outlined by Hoggett and Bishop, again illustrating that deaf people took part in leisure and sport for the same reasons as their hearing counterparts.[56]

Stewart shows that whilst deaf people become involved in sport for precisely the same reasons as hearing sportsmen, the audiological status of other competitors affects the types of benefits that can be gained. Whilst deaf sport caters more to the social needs of deaf sportsmen, hearing sport provides more 'physical gratification' because of the perception of hearing sport as being more skilful and of a better standard.[57] Lawson describes deaf sport as a means by which deaf people have formed 'a cohesive and mutually supportive community'.[58] Padden includes sport amongst the social factors which helped deaf people maintain contact with each other, and deaf sport regularly included a great deal of attendant socialisation. Sport has also acted as an entry route into the deaf community for those who are tentative about making a commitment to full membership: 'Sport offers deaf athletes an opportunity to test the social environment of the deaf community without fully adapting to its social and communicative demands'.[59] Deaf sport was also a way in which deaf clubs recruited new members. 'When I was younger, I wasn't interested in the deaf club, I thought it was boring, but then I followed my brothers into the football team and got involved [in the deaf club] that way'.[60] This was particularly important for younger deaf people who may have attended a deaf school far from their home and who had no contact with the local deaf community. 'You could go to someone's house and say, "I remember you from school. Do you want to come and join the deaf football club?" and they would say yes.[61]

It is clear that leisure and sport have long played an important role in helping to define communities and in providing community members with a sense of shared identity and cultural expression. For deaf club members, sharing leisure and sporting activities provided opportunities to find release from the stresses of daily life. This shared activity also allowed members to exercise a degree of choice over what they took part in and with whom. The deaf clubs served as an entry route into the social and cultural life of the deaf community, and members were able to find personal and shared identities. Deaf clubs and their social activities served an essential purpose in bringing new members into the community, particularly as there is no guaranteed entry route through family members. Leisure and sport were just as important in helping to maintain the deaf community as they have been in any other community group. In order to apply these arguments to a more detailed discussion of the role of leisure and sport within the deaf community, an analysis of the types and frequency of deaf people's leisure and sport activities is required. This is provided in the following chapters, based on the reported activities of deaf club members in the pages of *British Deaf News*, whose role in the deaf community is outlined next. A broad picture of deaf leisure across the United Kingdom leads into a detailed case study of north-west England. This will help illustrate not only the extent and variety of deaf leisure but also the important psychological and emotional rewards deaf people gained from the events themselves and from the notions of shared identity and community cohesion that were an equally important consequence of deaf leisure.

Notes

1   St John, W., 'Just what do we mean by community? Conceptualizations from the field', *Health and Social Care in the Community* 6, 2 (1998), pp. 63–70

2   Crow, G. and G.A. Allan, *Community life* (Hemel Hempstead: Harvester Wheatsheaf, 1994), p. 3

3   Meegan, R. and A. Mitchell, '"It's not community round here, it's neighbour-hood": neighbourhood change and cohesion in urban regeneration policies', *Urban Studies* 38, 12 (2001), pp. 2167–2194

4   Crow and Allan, *Community life*, p. 4

5   *Ibid.*

6   *Ibid.*, p. 3

7   Kyle and Woll, *Sign language*, p. 11

8   Loy, J.W. and G.S. Kenyon, *Sport, culture and society* (London: MacMillan, 1969) p. 15

9   Bishop, J. and P. Hoggett, 'Mutual aid in leisure' in C. Critcher, P. Bramham and A. Tomlinson (eds.), *Sociology of leisure: a reader* (London: Chapman and Hall, 1995), pp. 197–208

10   Padden, 'The deaf community and deaf culture'; Padden, 'The deaf community and the culture of deaf people'; Higgins, *Outsiders*

11   Bishop and Hoggett, 'Mutual aid in leisure', p. 201

12   *Ibid.*, p. 206

13   Crow and Allan, *Community life*, p. 4

14   Rose, P. and G. Kiger, 'Intergroup relations: political action and identity in the deaf community', *Disability and Society* 10, 4 (1995), p. 522

15   Bishop and Hoggett, 'Mutual aid in leisure', p. 198

16   Rose and Kiger, 'Intergroup relations', p. 552

17   Padden, 'The deaf community and deaf culture', p. 2

18   Shogan, D., 'Characterizing constraints of leisure: a Foucaultian analysis of leisure constraints', *Leisure Studies* 21 (2002), pp. 27–38

19   Devas, 'Support and access in sports'

20   Hodson interview

21   Padden and Humphries, *Deaf in America*, p. 49

22   Atherton, M., D. Russell and G.H. Turner, *Deaf United* (Coleford: Douglas McLean, 2000), p. 79

23   *Ibid.*

24   Metcalfe, A., 'Sport and community: a case study of the mining villages of East Northumberland, 1800–1914' in Hill and Williams, *Sport and identity*, p. 15

25   Morris, D., *The soccer tribe* (London: Cape, 1981), pp. 17–20

26   Lane, H., 'Why the deaf are angry' in Lee, *Deaf liberation*, pp. 121–135

27   Padden, 'The deaf community and deaf culture', p. 44. Examples relating to deaf sport are given in Atherton *et al.*, *Deaf United*, pp. 82–96

28   Peillon, M., 'Bourdieu's field and the sociology of welfare', *Journal of Social Policy* 27, 2 (1998), pp. 213–229

29   Dhesi, A.S., 'Social capital and community development', *Community Development Journal* 35, 3 (2000), pp. 199–214; A. Ward and G. Tampubolon, 'Social capital, networks and leisure consumption', *The Sociological Review* 50, 2 (2002) pp. 155–180

30   The social exclusion of deaf people in the workplace is discussed by Young *et al.*, *Looking on* and Montgomery and Laidlaw, *Occupational dissonance*

31   Peillon, 'Bourdieu's field', pp. 216–217

32   Puttnam, *Bowling alone*

33   Crow and Allan, *Community life*, p. 4; Bishop and Hoggett, 'Mutual aid in leisure', p. 206

34   Holt, *Sport and the British*, p. 347

35   MacClancy, *Sport, identity and ethnicity*, p. 2

36   Holt, *Sport and the British*, pp. 366–367

37   Wohl, A. and E. Pudelkiewicz, 'Theoretical and methodological assumptions of research on the processes of involvement in sport and sport socialization', *International Review of Sports Sociology* 7 (1972), pp. 69–84

38   Bishop and Hoggett, 'Mutual aid in leisure', p. 201

39   Jarvie, G. and J. Maguire, *Sport and leisure in social thought* (London: Routledge, 1994), pp. 9–10

40   Durkheim, E., *The division of labour* (London: Collier Macmillan, 1964)

41   Holt, *Sport and the British*, pp. 261–262

42   Puttnam, *Bowling alone*

43   Weiss, 'Identity reinforcement in sport'

44   *Ibid.*, p. 397

45   This information is drawn from an interview conducted by the author in 1997 for the *Deaf United* project. The informant's identity was concealed to preserve anonymity and remains so here. See Atherton *et al.*, *Deaf United*

46   Atherton *et al.*, *Deaf United*, p. 79

47   Tuan, *Topophilia*, p. 4

48   Bale, *Sport, space and the city*

49   Eyles, J., *Senses of place* (Warrington, Silverbrook, 1985)

50   Bale, *Sport, space and the city*, pp. 64–77

51   Wise, 'Home: territory and identity'

52   Ammons, D.K. and M.S. Miller, 'Sports, deafness and the family', in Erting, C. J. and R. Johnson, *The deaf way: perspectives from the international conference on deaf culture* (Washington DC: Gallaudet University Press, 1994), p. 542

53   Stewart, D., *The impact of sports within the deaf community* (Washington DC: Gallaudet University Press, 1993), p. 1

54   *Ibid.*, p. 2

55   Weiss, 'Identity reinforcement in sport', p. 397

56   Bishop and Hoggett, 'Mutual aid in leisure', p. 201

57   Stewart, *Deaf sports*, pp. 126–131; Atherton *et al.*, *Deaf United*, p. 73

58   Lawson, 'The role of sign', p. 32

59   Stewart, *Deaf sports*, p. 37

60   Atherton *et al.*, *Deaf United*, p. 17

61   *Ibid.*

5

BRITISH DEAF NEWS:
A WINDOW ON THE DEAF WORLD

The existence of a group of people who identify themselves as members of a distinct community based primarily on their shared deafness is without dispute. The members of this community are geographically dispersed; there are no places in Britain where the majority of inhabitants are deaf. However, it has been established that a locus for the community's activities was provided by the network of deaf clubs that were established from the mid-nineteenth century. In these clubs, deaf people were able to develop notions of identity based on mutual deafness and a communal form of social, cultural and linguistic expression. The cultural expression of this identity then served to strengthen and maintain the sense of community. These clubs would have remained to some extent isolated, self-contained communities without some means of maintaining regular contact and sharing information with each other. The main form for this communication was provided by a series of publications aimed at deaf people, the most recent of which is *British Deaf News (BDN)*. These newspapers and magazines allowed deaf people to keep abreast of events outside their own club by disseminating news across the British deaf community. Along with its immediate predecessor *British Deaf Times*, *BDN* provided the primary source of information about deaf people's social lives for this book. The titles included news on all aspects of deaf people's lives, and large sections of each issue were devoted to passing on information relating to the social activities of the various deaf clubs and their members from across the United Kingdom. Because of this, *BDN* provides a wealth of information on the social and leisure activities of deaf people.[1]

Newspapers are becoming an increasingly important source of data and information for cultural historians across a range of disciplines and interests, with stories, letters and editorials used to reconstruct history from the perspectives of both readers and publishers.[2] As Tunstall states, 'The press reflects

British history, and caricatures social divisions' and as such provides insights into a range of popular views and opinions.[3] Some examples of the ways newspapers have informed a variety of research topics include their value in tracing family histories, displaying attitudes to disadvantaged community groups, recording the impact of sporting events on sections of society, and in providing insights into the views and opinions expressed by letter writers to newspapers from earlier periods.[4] Another reason why printed materials such as newspapers are becoming increasingly important for academic research is that 'they are an important creator and transmitter of cultural values and ideas, and socio-political ideologies'.[5] Anderson highlights the importance of newspapers as a means of binding members of a community together, stating that each newspaper provides a connection between its readers, who could not otherwise come together in the same place at the same time. The development of 'print capitalism' is, he argues, an essential stage in the process of community consolidation.[6] Reading the same newspapers allows the large-scale transmission of these 'cultural values and ideas' and thus plays a part in developing the sense of belonging to a wider community described by Anderson as 'nationhood'. Newspapers are important in this process as they help to shape and inform opinions and create feelings of shared identity amongst their readers. However, the transmission of identity as performed by newspapers is not a one-way process. The way in which stories are reported can also be influenced by issues of identity that arise from the target readerships.[7] As well as creating and transmitting culturally defining information, newspapers record events and opinions that are derived from their readerships. On a number of geographical levels, whether local, regional or national, newspapers have to share an identity with their readers, by broadly reflecting the views and opinions of their target readership.[8] An analysis of newspaper content can therefore provide important insights into not only the lives of their readers, but also into what readers of particular titles believe in and aspire to. Newspapers can also act as an important supplement to official records, by providing examples and specific information that may not be included in the formal accounts kept by authorities or organisations. Official records are often statistically based, with totals, trends and aggregates being the main focus of what is recorded. In situations where specific examples of the events being recorded are needed, newspapers can provide this information and thus illustrate the bare statistics of official accounts. Local newspapers tend to focus more on community issues and 'human interest' stories, whilst national stories are often reported in terms of local impact.[9] National publications aimed at particular community groups operate in a similar way; although they may have a wider geographical focus, they share many of the characteristics of a local newspaper in the way stories are chosen and addressed.[10] In such titles, community membership is expressed through factors other than shared geographical location. In both types of paper, the readership acts as both the focus of the publication (by having community views and perspectives reported and reflected) and as the source of its content (by providing the topics and stories covered). In doing so, these publications inform and influence community members and help them, as readers of the newspaper, to share feelings of community with all other readers of the same paper. Using the example of the *London Evening Standard*, Glover shows that a local newspaper may be defined on more than merely geographical considerations; 'local' can instead be linked to shared interests amongst the paper's readers. '*The Evening Standard* has gone for the community of interest, rather than the geographical community. It looks at the world through the eyes of the London commuter.'[11] Replace '*The Evening Standard*' with '*British Deaf News*' and 'London commuters' with 'the deaf community' and this is precisely the role that *BDN* and its predecessors have filled within the British deaf community. This was particularly true before the advent of new technology such as email and textphones that allowed immediate communication between deaf people (especially sign language users) for the first time. Before then, *BDN* was often the only form of regular contact deaf people had with the wider deaf community outside their immediate deaf club.

Research by Peter Jackson has shown that *British Deaf News* developed from an amalgamation of two separate and long established lines of publications, which were themselves preceded by a number of earlier publications dating back over a number of years.[12]

Table 1 A genealogy of *British Deaf News*[13]

1889–1891 *Deaf and Dumb Times*	1905–1908 *Bolton and District Society Quarterly News*
1891–1892 *Deaf Chronicle*	1908–1909 *Quarterly News*
1892–1895 *British Deaf Mute* and *Deaf Mute Chronicle*	1909–1915 *Deaf Quarterly News* (Bolton)
1896–1903 *British Deaf Monthly*	1915–1950 *Deaf Quarterly News*
1903–1954 *British Deaf Times*	1950–1954 *Deaf News*
Titles merged in 1955 as *British Deaf News*	

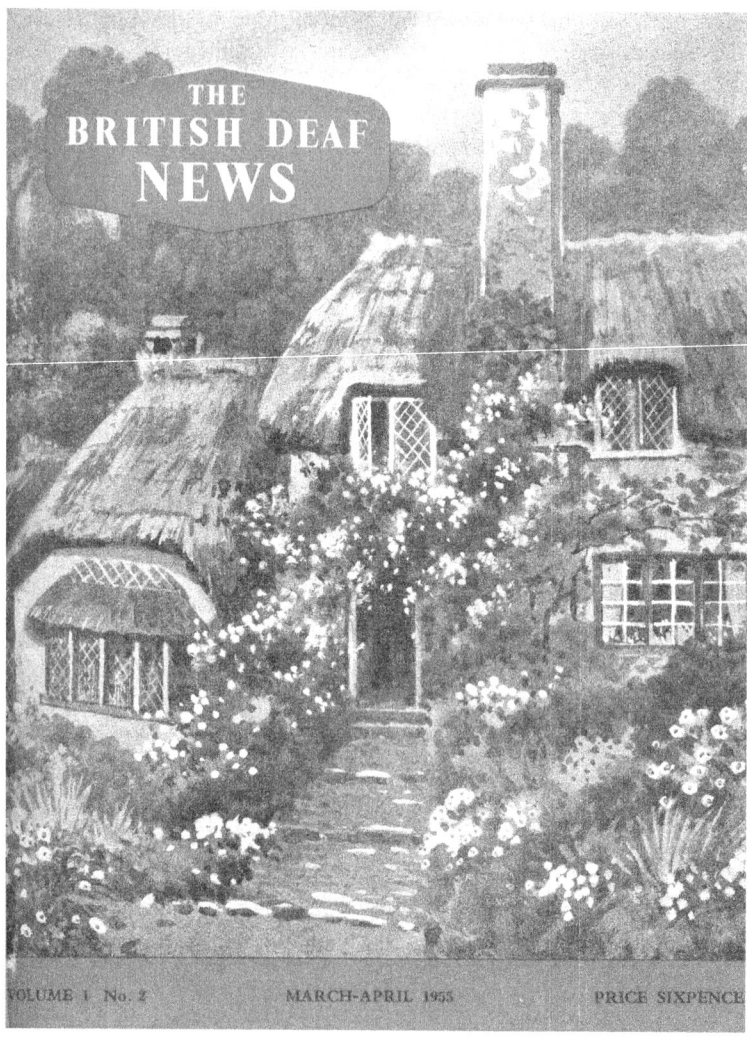

Figure 1 The cover of *British Deaf News* in 1955; the cosy imagery displayed here was a feature of the paper for many years

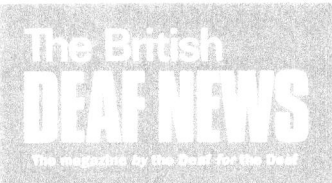

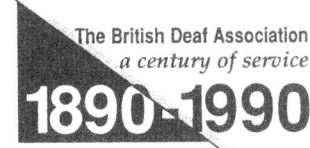

The British Deaf Association
a century of service
1890–1990

Major Victory on Broadcasting Bill

Deaf Accord (The British Association of the Hard of Hearing, The British Deaf Association, The National Deaf Children's Society, Sense, the National Deaf-Blind and Rubella Association and The National Deaf-Blind League) and the Deaf Broadcasting Council, claimed a major victory on 15th February as they welcomed the Government's announcement that the new Channel 3 and 5 licensees would be required to subtitle at least half of all their programmes within five years of the start of their franchises in 1993.

The announcement was made by Minister David Mellor at the end of a debate in the House of Commons.

"We are delighted that the Government has recognised the need to ensure the rights of deaf people in this way" said Jane Oberman, Parliamentary Officer of Deaf Accord. "We have been lobbying intensively on this issue over the last

few months, and have received widespread support from MPs from all parties for improved services".

Deaf people throughout the country had been contacting their MPs, and 150,000 signatures were collected on petitions which were presented to over 350 MPs, earlier in the year.

"These changes will mean that deaf people will have much more choice in what they can watch" said Austin Reeves from the Deaf Broadcasting Council, "but we are hoping that an obligation to include some programmes with sign language will be included at a later stage in the consideration of the Broadcasting Bill."

"British Sign Language is the first or only language of over 50,000 profoundly deaf people. It is a visual language that cannot be written down and having some daily news coverage in sign language would give this group of deaf people access to information that they are at present denied".

BDA launches 100th year celebrations

Special reports inside this issue:

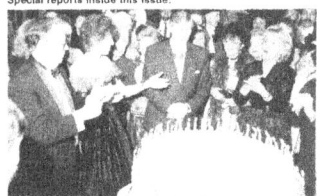

*Public launch by BDA Patron in London, page 3
*John Hay meets Lilian Lawson in Face to Face, pages 8&9
*Staff and Regional reports in BDA Office News, pages 10&11
*Special 4-page feature from Leeds in the BDA/Nat West Centenary Newsletter _free_ inside.

INSIDE: TWO YEARS AFTER GALLAUDET'S "DEAF PRESIDENT NOW" CAMPAIGN BDN TAKES ANOTHER LOOK, SEE PAGES 6&7

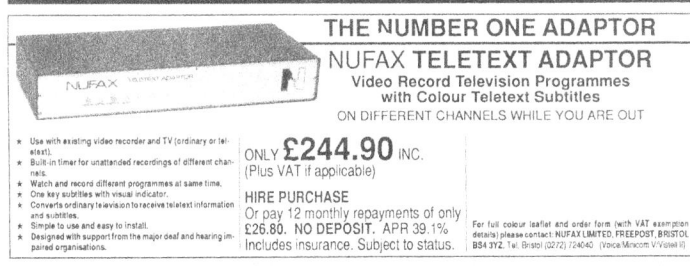
Figure 2 A more politically overt *BDN* cover from 1990, reflecting the growth in activism amongst deaf club members

British Deaf News was founded in 1955 when *British Deaf Times* and *Deaf News* merged into a single title, and acted as the main forum through which the British Deaf Association (BDA) could keep in touch with its members. As the above table illustrates, *BDN* was the successor to a number of periodicals aimed at deaf readers and others involved in the deaf world. The evidence provided by these and earlier deaf periodicals shows that groups of deaf people across Britain were using these publications to record and report their activities from at least the middle of the nineteenth century.[14] This history of newspapers aimed at deaf readers indicates that the deaf community, expressed as a group of people with shared outlooks, experiences and a common language, has been in existence for a significant period of time. These publications were pivotal in cementing the links between deaf people by acting as a medium for the circulation of information, news and opinions. The majority of these titles had close links to the various deaf organisations, most especially the BDA. Anderson's claim that newspapers are important elements in the development of ideas of community and nationhood is echoed by Brian Grant. He contends that 'the British Deaf Association and its activities have played a vital part in fostering the deaf community's identity and cohesion as a social group. The *British Deaf News* has been a cornerstone in this endeavour'.[15] By providing a means of regular contact between the national network of deaf clubs, *BDN* allowed its readers to feel part of a much wider community of deaf people.

BDN and its predecessors did not employ reporters, but instead relied for the majority of its content on a network of contributors across the country sending in stories, articles and news items concerning or involving deaf people. The essentially voluntary basis by which *BDN* gathered copy for publication illustrates the role the paper and its predecessors played within the community. Several of *BDN*'s forerunners folded because of financial pressures, but despite repeated failures, the table on the previous page shows that a new publication aimed at deaf readers always emerged. Rather than being a commercially driven venture, *BDN* was aimed at maintaining contact between deaf people. In essence, the paper was produced by the deaf community for the deaf community, rather than being primarily concerned with making a profit for its publishers. News concerning the activities of deaf clubs and their members, along with details of deaf sporting events, were provided by officials of the clubs and various deaf organisations. In this way, the content of *BDN* was not only directly relevant to its readers but also reflected issues and perspectives from within the heart of the community. In doing so, *BDN* constitutes a 'Newspaper of Record'; the paper provides not only information to its readers but a historical record of immense values to all those interested in the British deaf community.[16]

During the middle period of the twentieth century, deaf newspapers developed a format that was to remain largely unchanged until the very end of the century. Although providing national coverage, *BDN* acted essentially as a local newspaper for the deaf community, by focusing on issues from the point of view of deaf people. Fiske shows how such community-based reporting serves as a counterpoint to official or external views, and provides alternative perspectives from within the community.[17] So editions of the paper included reports of events in the hearing world that were related in some way to deafness or deaf people; news of new technology, such as telephones designed for deaf users; and legislation that affected deaf people. The human interest aspect of local newspapers was reflected by stories about deaf people from around the world ('Girdle around the World'), and the two central pillars of *BDN* for the first forty years of its existence, the 'Deaf Sport' and 'Around the clubs' pages. The 'Around the clubs' pages followed the format previously used in *British Deaf Times* until a change in publisher in 1999 saw the section finally dropped. Contributors brought news of the deaf clubs and their social and sporting activities to the attention of readers across Britain. Stories of interaction – and especially success – in and with the hearing world also featured regularly. Right up until the late 1980s, news of religious and church-based activities remained a regular and important element of the news passed on through these pages. Births, engagements and marriages also featured consistently, as did quite personal news about deaf club members suffering injury, accident, illness and death. Deaf people do not seem to have objected to this type of personal information being disseminated through *BDN*, as no apologies or letters of complaint were found in any of the issues investigated. This suggests that the 'gossip' element of these pages was accepted and even appreciated by deaf readers, allowing them the opportunity to keep up to date with friends and acquaintances across the country. By helping to keep deaf people in touch with one another's activities, *British Deaf News* showed itself to have an importance beyond that of a mere recorder and reporter of such news. It is because of its central role in both reporting and maintaining the deaf community that *British Deaf News* is such an essential and important source for any research into the lived experiences of deaf people, particularly deaf club members.

Deaf newspapers as a research resource

The quantitative data indicating the range and frequency of deaf club members' social activities presented in this book was derived from an analysis of *British Deaf Times* and *British Deaf News*. This analysis covered the period from 1945 to 1995, based on a full year's editions of the newspaper taken at five yearly intervals. The majority of the data collected was collated from the 'Around the Clubs' and 'Deaf Sport' pages of these publications, with eleven separate years covered by the data collection process. These data were used to provide the overview of deaf leisure outlined in chapter six and for the case study of north-west England provided in chapter eight. Data for 1945 and 1950 was drawn from *BDN*'s immediate predecessor, *British Deaf Times*, the format of which *BDN* largely adopted; *BDN* was the source used from 1955 onwards. For simplicity both publications are referred to in the text as *BDN* but each title is identified separately for reference purposes. Publication dates varied between monthly, bi-monthly and quarterly throughout the research period, producing a total of eighty-six issues for analysis.

Data was grouped under headings that reflect the types of activities reported in *British Deaf News*. Data was arranged according to the years in which reports appeared in *BDN*, which is not necessarily the same year in which events took place. Because news was provided on a voluntary basis, there is some incon-sistency or delay in the contributions from various clubs at certain times. Occasionally, reports commence with phrases such as 'Apologies for not sending any news for a while' or 'Not much has been happening in our club recently'. This meant that not all the events included in the club news pages took place in the same calendar year as the newspaper was published. For example, Ashton-under-Lyne Deaf Club's 1989 Bonfire Night party was not reported until the March 1990 issue of *BDN*.[18] For consistency, it is the year of publication that was used in the analysis and reporting of events. Care also had to be exercised when recording sporting events, in order to avoid misrep-resenting the number of events that took place. For example, participation in a league or knock-out competition sometimes resulted in multiple reports as the season progressed. In such instances, it was involvement in the compe-tition that was recorded rather than the number of actual reports. This also serves as a useful reminder that despite the extensive detail that can be drawn from *BDN*, the way in which the newspaper gathered and recorded the various activities of deaf people means that only a partial view of deaf leisure activity can be reconstructed. It must therefore be acknowledged that there was much more going on in terms of deaf people's leisure lives than merely that reported in *BDN*.

Nevertheless, *BDN* provides a useful insight into deaf life, its patterns and changes, and the wide range of activities deaf people engaged in during the years under investigation. The 'Around the clubs' feature listed the activities of the numerous deaf clubs and their members, whilst the 'Deaf Sport' pages offered information on the types of sporting activities deaf people chose to take part in, and with whom. As a research resource, *BDN* provides a national picture of the social lives of members of the deaf community, the prevalent views expressed by and towards the deaf community, and the various facets of what might be termed 'the deaf experience'. The breadth and detail of the data provided through these reports offers extensive information from which to identify types and patterns of activity. The extent and quality of the information available from *British Deaf News* makes it the most detailed and extensive record on which to base any quantitative and detailed research into the social lives of ordinary deaf people. Without the insights into the deaf world provided by *British Deaf News* and its predecessors, the research conducted for this book could not have been as thorough or as widely representative of the full range of deaf leisure experiences as it is.

One reason for making such a bold statement is that there are a number of problems with attempting to use other potential sources of primary information. Although deaf clubs were run on a formal basis, with committees and elected officers, it was not possible to identify any clubs with records covering the whole or majority of the years of this research. Even when the existence of official club records was confirmed, the available material is largely incomplete and access was not necessarily possible. If it had been possible to reconstruct the formal business of a particular club, it is questionable how useful this would be in assisting a qualitative study of the social lives of deaf club members. Nor could such an example be guaranteed to be wholly representative of the way deaf clubs across north-west England (the case study for this research) took decisions relating to their leisure activities. Across the country as a whole, deaf club records cannot match the breadth and depth of coverage given by *BDN*. Although the picture painted by *BDN* is not complete, it is nevertheless more comprehensive than any other available written source and provides significant amounts of direct evidence from those involved. The other potential source for direct primary evidence would have been to interview deaf club members. However, this too presents problems. For example, attempting to interview participants involved in activities that occurred during the 1940s or 1950s would be extremely unlikely to be successful sixty or seventy years after the event. Finding those involved in any event, not matter how comparatively recent, would present significant practical difficulties for an uncertain outcome. Recording and reporting any interviews pose certain logistical problems, but these are not insurmountable.[19] However, the question of the accuracy of data drawn from personal memory over such a long period of time would remain. The advantage of using the club pages of *BDN* is that these offer an alternative form of oral testimony and this testimony was produced soon after the events, whilst memory, enjoyment and other factors were still fresh in the minds of those reporting the activities. The pages of *BDN* thus act as a permanently accessible and constant record on the life of the deaf community, produced by those with direct involvement in the events.

The data gathered will be described in detail in subsequent chapters, but a brief indication of some of the findings serves to illustrate the value of *BDN* as a research source. The social and sporting news pages of *British Deaf News* indicate what news and information deaf club members felt was important to pass on to other deaf people. In doing so, the 'Around the Clubs' and 'Deaf Sport' pages add an important qualitative element to the quantitative information that can be gleaned from this source, indicating those aspects of their social lives deaf people themselves attached comparative value and importance to. From this information, some understanding of the motivations of deaf people in choosing to take part in certain activities can be gained. In addition, this information often contradicts some of the notions and stereotypes discussed previously that are applied to the deaf community – both from outside and from within the community itself. The news contained in *BDN* shows that far from being isolated or disabled because of their deafness, many profoundly deaf people were taking part in a wide range of activities, with both deaf and hearing people, as individuals and in groups of varying sizes. For example, the details of holidays taken by deaf people in groups and as individuals show that deaf people were no less adventurous or more restricted than their hearing neighbours. Trips throughout Europe were common from the 1960s onwards, and groups of deaf people were often to be found in many exotic or unexpected places. Examples include Liverpool Deaf Club members making a trip to Oberammergau in 1960 to watch the Passion Play, whilst a group of 120 deaf people from Preston went on a Caribbean cruise in 1975.[20]

News of club activities also provides information that is both unexpected and illuminating, and which challenges some of the existing conceptions of the nature of the deaf community and the way it chooses to enjoy itself. It might be presumed that the majority of deaf club members would have no interest in sound-based entertainments such as music. They were after all deaf. However, *British Deaf News* reported in 1965 that the younger members of Liverpool Deaf Club had been entertained at their Christmas party by what was described as 'a beat group'. Rory Storm and the Hurricanes – a well known group at the time and famous for being the group Ringo Starr left to join the Beatles – were the guests and proved to be so popular that the club intended booking similar groups in the near future. Indeed, the Dee Jays performed at the deaf club a few weeks later.[21] The reports mention that suitable amplification was provided; illustrating that not all deaf leisure activity was necessarily silent by nature. As was shown earlier, sign language was the main form of communication within the deaf clubs. However, the news pages show that many deaf clubs also had what were termed 'Hard of Hearing' sections. This indicates that some clubs were prepared to include all deaf people, not merely sign language users. There is further evidence that questions just how deaf some deaf club members were. In one example, a group of deaf people from Bolton Deaf Club attended a show at Manchester's Palace Theatre featuring the comedians Morecambe and Wise, but no mention is made of an interpreter being present, and it is extremely unlikely one would have been provided in those far-off days. [22] This then raises questions about how the deaf members of the audience followed what was happening on stage, and the reasons behind the decision to attend. These issues will be discussed in more detail later, but this example serves as an illustration of the type of qualitative questions that arise from the quantitative data available from *British Deaf News*.

These examples underline the value and validity of *British Deaf News* as a primary source of data on deaf social activity. All members of the deaf community were included, with reports quite literally covering all events from 'the cradle to the grave'. In effect, the club news sections of *BDN* acted largely as a collection of human interest stories that were interesting and relevant to deaf people. *British Deaf News*, as the de facto local newspaper of the deaf community, shares the 'advantage of being first and arguably best in their reportage of local stories' that McNair claims is an important feature of local and regional press. [23] As such, *BDN* provides a detailed insight into communal deaf social life that cannot be gained from any other recorded source.

Notes

1 Deaf people use the acronym *BDN* for *British Deaf News* and this is used throughout this book for both *British Deaf Times* and *British Deaf News*, particularly as the majority of data was drawn from the latter publication. However, footnote references to specific issues of these newspapers will be given as either *BDT* or *BDN* as appropriate

2 Tunstall, J., *The media in Britain* (London: Constable, 1983), B. Popik , 'Digital historical newspapers: a review of the powerful new research tools', *Journal of English Linguistics* 32, 2 (2004), pp. 114–123 and J. Campbell, 'Why papers of record are history', *British Journalism Review* 17, 59 (2006), pp. 59–64

3 Tunstall, *The media in Britain*, p. 75

4 Examples include E. McLaughlin, *Family history from newspapers* (Aylesbury, Varneys, 1994); N. Gold and G. Auslander, 'Newspaper coverage of people with disabilities in Canada and Israel: an international comparison', *Disability and Society* 14, 6, (1999), pp. 709–731; John Harris, 'Lie back and think of England: the women of Euro 96', *Journal of Sport and Social Issues*, 23, 1 (1999) pp. 96–110; P. Farrer, *Men in petticoats: a selection of letters from Victorian newspapers* (London: Karn, 1987)

5   Soothill, K. and C. Grover, 'A note on computer searches of newspapers' *Sociology* 31, 3 (1997), p. 591

6   Anderson, *Imagined communities*, pp. 35–40

7   For examples, see L. Connell, 'The Scottishness of the Scottish press: 1918–1939' *Media, Culture and Society* 25 (2003), pp. 187–207; W. Bokhorst-Heng, 'Newspapers in Singapore: a mass ceremony in the imagining of the nation', *Media, Culture and Society* 24, 4 (2002), pp. 559–569

8   Law, A., 'Near and far: banal national identity and the press in Scotland', *Media, Culture and Society* 23, (2003), p. 300

9   Aldridge, M., 'The ties that divide: regional press campaigns, community and populism', *Media, Culture and Society* 25, (2003), pp. 491–509; R. Pilling, 'The changing role of the local journalist: from faithful chronicler of the parish pump to multiskilled compiler of an electronic database' in B. Franklin and D. Murphy (eds), *Making the local news: local journalism in context* (London: Routledge, 1998), pp. 183–195

10 Examples include *The Voice, Gay News* and *The Jewish Chronicle*

11 Glover, M., 'Looking at the world through the eyes of ...: reporting the "local" in daily, weekly and Sunday local newspapers' in B. Franklin and D. Murphy (eds), *Making the local news: local journalism in context* (London: Routledge, 1998), p. 119

12 Jackson, P., *Britain's deaf heritage* (Edinburgh: Pentland, 1990), pp. 279–282

13 Based on a diagram in Jackson, *Britain's deaf heritage,* p. 280

14 Jackson (*Britain's deaf heritage*, p. 279) cites 1843 as the year in which the first deaf newspaper was established in Edinburgh

15 Grant, *Deaf advance*, p. 120

16 Campbell, J., *British Journalism Review*, pp. 59–64

17 Fiske, J., 'Popularity and the politics of information' in P. Dahlgren and C. Sparks (eds), *Journalism and popular culture* (London: Sage, 1992), pp. 45–63

18 *BDN*, 1990 March, p. 13

19 Recording interviews with sign language users are discussed in M. Atherton, D. Russell and G.H. Turner, 'Looking to the past: the role of oral history research in recording the visual history of Britain's deaf community', *Oral History* 29, 2 (2001), pp. 35–47

20 *BDN*, 1960, p. 63; 1975, p. 28

21 *BDN*, 1965, p. 255

22 *BDN*, 1965, p. 251

23 McNair, B., *News and journalism in the UK* (London: Routledge, 2003), p. 207

6

COMMUNAL DEAF LEISURE IN
POST-WAR BRITAIN

Evidence drawn from deaf newspapers shows that much of the social life of deaf people was communal in nature, it involved the presence of other deaf people and was centred on the deaf clubs. This continued a tradition of participation and choice in recreation activities that dated back to before the Second World War. However, these activities were not solely restricted to the physical premises of the deaf club nor to events that only involved other deaf people. Deaf club members' activities were influenced by what was taking place in the outside world and regularly involved interaction with their hearing counterparts. Factors which affected deaf leisure included regional preferences for certain activities (especially sports), economic factors brought about by changes in industry and commerce, and broader trends and changes in the social life of the nation. How these factors impacted on deaf people's leisure lives across the UK will be the focus of this chapter.

The evidence gathered from *British Deaf News* demonstrates the range and frequency of the leisure activities deaf club members engaged in, both as individuals and collectively. As this chapter will show, deaf clubs were found across Great Britain and they provided and organised a variety of leisure and sporting events for their members. In addition, deaf clubs served as the preferred location for family gatherings and celebrations in which the wider deaf community, as represented by the clubs' members, were welcome and willing participants. What follows is a brief overview of deaf leisure, based on the reports published in *British Deaf News*. It is not possible to reconstruct an exhaustive or comprehensive record of all aspects of deaf leisure, as *BDN* only provides a snapshot of deaf clubs' activities and those of their members. Even so, the sheer volume of reports found in *BDN* makes a detailed analysis virtually impossible on a national scale, hence the case study of north-west England which follows later in this book. Although only based on a five yearly sample, the north-west region alone provides over two thousand reports of events and activities taking place in and through the region's deaf clubs; when extended across the country this figure rises to over twenty thousand reported events and activities. Even without a minute level of analysis, these data provide important insights into the particular types of deaf leisure and sport that reflect both the choices made by deaf people and their motivations in choosing certain activities and pastimes over others. This in turn allows greater insights into the everyday leisure lives of deaf club members and the importance of the services and events the clubs provided in maintaining and promoting the cohesiveness of the deaf community. So just how many of these deaf clubs were there in post-war Britain and where were they to be found?

Deaf clubs in Great Britain

As well as the 'Around the Clubs' pages, issues of *BDN* included a list of deaf clubs, missions and institutes right up until the early 1990s. From these two sources, it is possible to identify both the number and location of deaf clubs that were in existence between 1945 and 1995. In all, 242 clubs were found, covering all areas of the UK from the far north of Scotland to the farthest extremities of England and Wales. Whilst not all of these were in existence throughout the research period, there was a steady growth in their numbers from 1945 right up until 1990. Whilst some clubs closed down, they were often replaced by new ventures in the same or nearby towns. From 1990 onwards, the first signs of large-scale decline are evident and a number of closures occurred, with clubs merging or disappearing completely as younger deaf people found alternative venues for meeting. One example is Gosport Deaf Club on the Isle of Wight that closed down in 1990 after only three people attended the Annual General Meeting.[1] In the years since 1995 (the end of this study's focus period) the spiral of decline and closure has increased to the point where it is unlikely many will survive for much longer. The reasons for this gloomy outlook are discussed in the concluding chapter.

   Virtually every major town and city in the United Kingdom had at least one deaf club, with larger cities often having more, sometimes representing different religious backgrounds. For the purposes of this analysis, these deaf clubs were allocated to one of eleven regions from across mainland Great Britain. This closely follows the pattern of organisation of the British Deaf Association, which had a similar number of regional councils during the period covered by this study.

Table 2 The distribution of deaf clubs across Britain

Region	No. of deaf clubs
Scotland	21
North west	28
North east	18
Yorkshire	14
West Midlands	13
East Midlands and Lincolnshire	14
Wales and North Midlands	24
South west	21
London and South east	50
East Anglia and Home counties	23
South coast	16

As this table clearly indicates, deaf clubs were not restricted to certain areas of the country. The clubs ranged from a few people meeting in a local vicarage for bible reading classes to the multiple clubs in places such as London, Birmingham and Manchester that catered for a larger local deaf population. Their higher membership numbers are often reflected in a greater number of events being organised and reported in *British Deaf News*, but even the smaller clubs served an important social function for deaf people.

Not surprisingly the greatest concentration of clubs was found in London, but even comparatively small towns such as Blyth in Northumberland, Crewkerne in Somerset and St Leonards in Kent all had their own deaf clubs. Wales was served by eighteen deaf clubs, with many of these serving small local deaf populations in places such as Hengoed, Pontlottyn and Llanberis. Although somewhat isolated geographically and almost certainly only having a few members, the presence of deaf clubs in such places emphasises the importance of being able to meet up with other deaf people; this was after all the main reason for the clubs' existence as they emerged as the social aims of voluntary welfare organisations. Members of all deaf clubs, whether large or small, had access to a range of leisure activities and consequently a much wider social circle and a more extensive community of deaf people than merely the members of their own club. In the larger urban centres, these networks were sometimes constituted into a formal association, such as the London Federation of Deaf Clubs, which promoted interaction and engagement between deaf clubs in the capital. Deaf sport was similarly organised into various regional bodies who arranged leagues and competitions involving their member clubs. Outside the cities, such ties were more informally organised but whether formalised or *ad hoc*, there was a wide range of leisure activities taking place in and through the deaf clubs.

The range of deaf communal leisure activities

The first thing to note about deaf people's leisure activities was that these were essentially the same as those of the hearing world. Deaf people were not spending their leisure time in ways that were markedly different from their hearing counterparts. What was different and which will be highlighted here in and in later chapters, is the way leisure activities were vital in establishing and nurturing a sense of community based on shared experiences of deafness. For the majority of deaf people, membership and involvement in a deaf club was not just one aspect of their leisure lives; it was often their sole form of rewarding social interaction, which was otherwise absent from their daily lives.

For the purposes of this study, the leisure activities reported in *British Deaf News* were grouped into eleven main headings; involvement in sport is dealt with separately.

Table 3 The recorded leisure activities of deaf club members

Dances and parties	Fundraising events
Trips and holidays	Church and religious events
Anniversaries and presentations	Community events
OAP events	Societies and courses
Youth and children events	Cards
Practical demonstrations and talks	

Particular examples of deaf club members' involvement in these activities will be examined in the case study of north-west England that follows later, but some general comments provide insights into precisely what deaf leisure involved. By far the most popular activity was going on trips and holidays, which could range from a trip to another deaf club in the area for an evening of bingo, darts, snooker and cards to a large scale communal holiday in Britain or even abroad. Two hundred and fifty deaf people from across the country travelling to Skegness in 1975 for a holiday organised by the British Deaf Association was just one of a number of such holidays that took place throughout the 1970s and 1980s.[2] Trips were not just restricted to Britain, with

Oxford Deaf Club being one of many to enjoy reciprocal visits with European deaf clubs, in this instance Bonn in West Germany. Oxford's exchange visits, which began in 1976, were still being reported in 1990, indicating these were not merely one-off occurrences.[3] Some deaf travellers were even more adventurous, as an admittedly extreme example from 1975 illustrates. Riding low-powered 50cc Honda mopeds and with their camping equipment strapped to the sides, three deaf club members from Devon set off to cross Europe. Despite numerous breakdowns and accidents (several before they had even crossed the Channel), they nevertheless managed to travel over 2,000 miles on a round trip that included Austria, Czechoslovakia, Poland and East Germany (these last three being communist countries at the time) as well as several brushes with Customs officials and police officers in each country.[4] Apparently the three friends were seasoned European travellers but this was their first venture into the eastern half of the continent and they saw nothing unusual in their trip.

Whilst more mundane visits between clubs remained a constant feature of deaf leisure life throughout the second half of the twentieth century, the venues for holidays became increasingly exotic as the century progressed. This reflected changing trends in wider society, as overseas holidays became ever more popular and affordable through increased disposable income, but it also helps to illustrate that deafness does not necessarily or automatically result in social isolation or a restricted social life. So by 1990, *BDN* was advertising holidays in Las Vegas, Hollywood and Orlando, which ranged in cost from £800 upwards for fourteen days; a significant sum at the time. The advertiser claimed to be 'the country's only specialist travel agency for the deaf and hearing impaired' with a range of holidays across Europe and further afield.[5] Rhodes was the preferred destination for a group of forty deaf people in 1990, whose two-week visit to the Greek island was accompanied by a sign language interpreter. Although days out and even communal holidays were a feature of many types of social club, the sheer regularity and diversity of those enjoyed by deaf club members marks this as one of the defining features of deaf leisure. Another important aspect of all deaf club outings, whether just a day trip or a longer overseas holiday, is that virtually all these events included contact with local deaf people. A day trip in Britain almost always involved calling in at a deaf club at some point, often in the evening for a social gathering, whilst trips such as that made by the deaf motorcyclists included visiting deaf clubs and even staying with deaf people in the countries on their itinerary. Such trips demonstrate that the term 'deaf club' had broader connotations than merely a place or a building; membership of a deaf club represented an attachment to a group of people and their shared values and ideals (that is to say active involvement in the deaf community) that was not dependent on any particular venue. It was the people involved in such events that embodied the concept of the deaf club, not necessarily the location – even when visiting another country.

However, the deaf club as a place was significant to its members, as is evidenced by the wide range of family events that were celebrated within the deaf clubs' premises. Virtually every important milestone in the lives of deaf club members (and often their families, whether deaf or hearing) was marked by a gathering to which many if not all other members were invited. Christenings, birthdays, engagements, weddings, anniversaries of all kinds and even funerals and wakes were all held in the deaf clubs and reported in the pages of *British Deaf News*. As well as family events, deaf clubs were also keen to arrange parties almost at the drop of a hat for a wide variety of reasons. Christmas parties for children and old age pensioners, summer fairs, fancy dress events, annual dinners and dances all formed part of the calendar of events for clubs across the country. These were also an important element of each club's fundraising efforts, which every club had to engage in to some extent. Deaf clubs were at least partially (if not wholly) self-financing and so a range of events were held to pay for regular items such as redecorating, purchasing new equipment or providing holidays for older or disabled members, as well as for special events. The rise in sponsored fundraising through the 1960s and 1970s was taken up by deaf clubs, who often adapted these events to reflect their particular interests and abilities. So as well as taking part in walks, cycle rides and pram pushes just as their hearing contemporaries did, some clubs had sponsored 'finger spelling' events for children and non-signing days for adults (a deaf alternative to a sponsored silence).[6] Later in the century a subtle change can be seen in the motivations behind deaf people's moneymaking ventures. As well as continuing to be the recipients of what were essentially charitable donations, deaf clubs began raising money for others. Early examples include children in various deaf clubs raising money for the annual Blue Peter appeal organised by the popular BBC Television children's programme and these were followed by events intended to raise funds for a range of local and national charities and appeals.[7]

One activity that was not reported in *British Deaf News* but which nevertheless was a staple element of deaf club life was bingo. Played in virtually every club, in an echo of other types of social club across the UK, bingo was adapted for play in a visual format, with the fundraising efforts of some larger clubs being directed to providing large display screens to identify the numbers called. The game was as much a part of club life as drinking and gossiping and so was very rarely mentioned. Playing various card games was equally popular but as they formed part of the highly competitive indoor sports programmes, this particular pastime was reported, especially when some notable feat was achieved, such as success in a local cards league.

The broader social purpose of deaf clubs

As well as being places of entertainment, deaf clubs increasingly became centres of education and information during the second half of the twentieth century. Many clubs held regular information sessions for their members, such as when decimal currency was introduced in 1969 or in the run-up to local and national elections. The introduction of various welfare provisions for deaf and disabled people in the 1990s saw many Benefits Agency officers visiting the clubs to explain deaf people's rights to various government funds. Courses for members were also run by or in the deaf clubs, with flower arranging, photography and calligraphy being popular right up until the 1990s. Practical courses in dressmaking and decorating could also be found across the country, whilst Fife Police put on a safe driving course for deaf people in 1970. Deaf clubs began to reach out to the wider community by starting to run sign language courses (which provided both employment for members and a useful source of income for both clubs and their members) from the 1980s.[8] As part of this venture, deaf awareness events were also held in local shopping centres, to raise the profile of deaf people amongst the general population and to challenge stereotypical views of deafness.

Engagement with the wider population was a feature of deaf leisure throughout the post-war period, but this often had charitable connotations. Voluntary groups such as the Lions, Round Table, Soroptimists and Freemasons were regular visitors to deaf clubs as well as hosting various joint events at their own venues. These often involved the charity making a donation of money or equipment to the local deaf club, which sometimes had conflicting consequences. On the one hand, deaf clubs received much needed financial help in the form of funds or equipment, but on the other these donations did not sit well with the arguments of deaf people themselves that deafness was not a disability and deaf people did not want to be seen as worthy of charity. Even so, *BDN* does not contain any reports of such assistance being refused; instead fundraising events – both for deaf clubs and other causes – became increasingly integrated affairs later in the century, with deaf people becoming active participants rather than merely the recipients of these efforts.

The close links between religious groups, most notably the Church of England, and deaf clubs was still evident in the post-war years. Many deaf clubs and societies met in church halls and had local clergymen as their nominal or actual leaders, and attendance at religious events still played an important part in many clubs' social calendars. This is most notable in the rise of signing choirs during the 1980s, with regional and national championships being established in response to the growing numbers of deaf choirs.[9] Deaf choirs

perform hymns and suitable secular songs in sign language, usually accompanied by a sung or recorded version, in an interesting adaptation of what might
be termed 'hearing culture'. Many churches also provided interpreted services
for their deaf congregations, with deaf people often travelling long distances to
attend. So whilst other aspects of communal deaf leisure went into decline, and
despite a gradual reduction in religious observance amongst the population
as a whole, organised religion still played a role in deaf life and leisure as the
twentieth century drew to a close.

Sport in the deaf clubs

In addition to recording deaf people's leisure activity, *British Deaf News*
reported the sporting activities of deaf club members, both as participants and
spectators. These data illustrate that sport has played an important part in the
lives of deaf club members for many years. However, the range of sports organised through the deaf clubs and the various deaf sporting bodies was somewhat
restricted, as will be discussed shortly.

Deaf sport was not formally organised at either regional or national levels
until the mid-twentieth century. Although a team of deaf sportsmen and
women represented Great Britain at the Silent Games of 1924 (the first international deaf sports competition), there was no national body overseeing
deaf sport until the formation of the British Deaf Amateur Sports Association
(BDASA) in 1930. In terms of European deaf sport, Britain lagged behind
countries such as Germany (1910), Sweden (1913) and France (1918) in
establishing a national governing body.[10] The BDASA was a purely voluntary organisation until 1982, arranging a number of competitions in various
sports at both regional and national levels. National competitions were usually
conducted on a regional basis initially, with the victorious teams then progress-
ing to a further competition to determine the national champions. By 1980,
the British Deaf Amateur Sports Association had become the British Deaf
Sports Council (BDSC), and the British Deaf Association (BDA) assumed
formal responsibility for funding deaf sports administration in 1982. The
BDSC became an affiliated member organisation of the BDA but retained its
autonomy. Roland Haythornthwaite became the BDSC's first paid employee;
previously the unpaid voluntary administrator of deaf sport, he became the
BDA's full-time Sports and Leisure Officer. The remainder of the BDSC's posts
continued to be manned by volunteers, with funding derived from donations
and the fundraising efforts of deaf club members.[11] In its heyday, the BDASA
had many thousands of members and at the time of the fiftieth anniversary
of organised deaf sport in Britain, there were reportedly over 8,500 members

involved in the sporting life of 120 deaf clubs, spread across eleven regional councils.[12] During the post-war years, a number of governing bodies for individual deaf sports emerged, usually but not exclusively operating under the aegis of the BDASA and its successor the BDSC. The number of deaf clubs in London made a local deaf sporting competition viable, as it did in the north-west but both the Federation of London Deaf Clubs (FLDC) and the Orme League in Lancashire were limited to the same few sports.

Deaf club based sport was largely restricted to football and indoor sports in winter whilst bowls and some limited participation in cricket filled the summer months. However, the majority of deaf sport has always been in competition with and against hearing sportsmen, rather than as 'deaf against deaf'.[13] Deaf football teams played more matches against hearing opponents than deaf ones and deaf bowlers were to be found playing in both crown green and flat bowls leagues across the country. Even in the most popular outdoor winter sport, finding adequate numbers of players and the costs of travelling across the country have mitigated against a national deaf football league. A league competition was established in the early 1980s but soon failed due to the expense of clubs having to travel long distances to fulfil fixtures. Instead, the main deaf football competition has remained the British Deaf Cup, an annual knock-out competition first established in 1928.[14]

Cricket in summer has been even more problematic, with the cricket club based at Lewisham Deaf Club in south-east London (founded in 1977) providing a rare example of a deaf team regularly playing together. A by-product of the highly successful football club wanting to spend their summers together, the cricket team repeated their winter activities by mostly playing against hearing teams. However, there were sufficient deaf cricket teams for a short-lived and small-scale FLDC championship to be held from 1977 to 1979 but this is the only post-war example of a deaf cricket league found in *BDN*.[15] The only other evidence found was of occasional one-off friendly matches played between deaf clubs but these were few and far between, with cricket not featuring prominently as a sport for deaf people. Bowls was much more popular, with regional variations amongst deaf people being determined by local preferences for crown green bowls in north-west England or flat green in other parts of the country. Deaf teams played in hearing leagues and both teams and individuals achieved degrees of success in winning leagues and cups. Interestingly, despite the popularity of the game and the numbers of deaf club members taking part, there were very few deaf-only bowls competitions reported in *British Deaf News*. Why this might be is not clear, but it is possible that, as deaf footballers have reported, playing with and against hearing players was seen as representing a higher standard of competition, even if it was less socially rewarding.[16] Swimming galas and athletics meetings also took place, but these were restricted to the regional and national championships organised by the British Deaf Sports Council.

There were often insufficient numbers of deaf people in a particular region of the country to support collective deaf involvement in a large number of sports, even in areas of the country where a particular sport was very popular. Thus there were no deaf rugby union competitions to be found in Wales or the west country, although there were a very few teams, and occasionally individual deaf players joined hearing teams. One notable anomaly is golf; whilst deaf people have been keen players of the game and have taken up the game in some numbers, they did so as individuals rather than as representatives of their deaf clubs. Although competitions for deaf golfers were held in certain parts of the country (but by no means all), these are the only examples of teams of deaf golfers and these are deaf-only contests. Deaf golfers do not appear to have played against hearing players to any great extent, even as individuals, perhaps indicating that communication barriers made 'mixed' golf less appealing due to the resulting lack of social rewards. Squash is another sport in which deaf people have reached high levels of skill and achievement but overall participation rates remained low, again raising questions about the influence of the non-sporting benefits that might be absent for deaf players. In both sports there has also been a marked regional preference, with most of those taking part coming from southern England, together with Scotland in the case of golf. The reasons for this lack of national participation are addressed in the case study of north-west England which follows later.

Indoor sports were even more popular than football as the main winter sporting pastime for deaf people, not least because a greater range of ages could take part. Consisting of various combinations of darts, cards, snooker, billiards and pool, with skittles and shove ha'penny featuring in southern England, indoor sports were one of the most important means by which the various sections of the deaf community maintained their links during the winter months. Clubs would travel to their local rivals for a weekly round of competition, food and socialising, and it is interesting to speculate on what the primary reason for the event taking place might have been. The opportunities for contact with other deaf people were almost certainly as psychologically rewarding as the sporting contests themselves, with many of those attending possibly having little interest in the sports but relishing the chance to meet old and new friends. The same was true of all sporting events and the social nature of sport contests between deaf people is evident in the staging of a party, disco or dinner dance after virtually every sporting event, whether a major competition or just a football match between two deaf clubs. As many deaf people reported in relation to their participation in football, whilst playing with and against hearing players offered the chance to play at a higher level, being a member of a deaf team and playing against deaf opponents brought greater social rewards. [17] For deaf people, such sporting events were as often an excuse to get together as they were to seek sporting success.

Why such a narrow range of deaf participation in sport?

It must be accepted that the extent of sporting activity reported in *BDN* was almost certainly incomplete, but nevertheless it is possible to gain a general overview of the degree of deaf sporting participation. From this, it is possible to draw some broad conclusions concerning the involvement of deaf people in various sports, with and against both deaf and hearing opponents. It is clear from the amount of space devoted to the subject in *British Deaf News* that sport played a major role in the broader social and leisure activities of deaf club members during the post-war period. The evidence available from *BDN* shows that there were significant numbers of deaf people enjoying a variety of sporting activities across the UK between 1945 and 1995. In this, deaf people showed themselves to be no different to the rest of the population. Just as in the hearing world, there were some regional variations in terms of the sports engaged in and some sports experienced periods of popularity and decline, but the overall picture is of a group of people who were regularly brought together for and by their enjoyment of sporting contests. Deaf people not only played against each other, but they also engaged – as groups and as individuals – with hearing people as teammates and opponents. However, despite the levels of activity, the range of deaf sporting activity was somewhat narrow. Only eleven distinct sports were reported with any degree of regularity throughout the fifty years covered by this study. Others may have featured very occasionally, but the evidence indicates that the eleven sports included in this analysis represent the main sporting pastimes of deaf club members. Many competitive pastimes which were enjoyed and actively pursued by other social and community groups, such as pigeon racing or angling, do not appear to have featured in the organised sporting activity of the deaf clubs. If they were included, then this participation was not reported in *BDN*. Sports that were popular with deaf people in some parts of the country, such as squash and golf, were not enjoyed more widely by deaf people across Britain.

One factor in the choices deaf people made about their involvement with certain sports may be linked to social class. Wilson argues that social class can be an important factor in involvement in sport generally and more specifically the types of sports a particular group or class chooses to pursue. The more working-class a social group, the more restricted the types of sports they will be involved in. [18] Wilson refers to those sports followed by the working class as 'prole' sports, which can include such sports as football, snooker, bowls and darts. Whilst these 'prole' sports represent those most popular amongst deaf club members across the UK, this does not necessarily mean that all deaf people's sporting participation was restricted to those sports most often associated with the working class. Sports not traditionally associated with the working class such as table tennis and netball were occasionally reported in various parts of Britain. Deaf people were also quite possibly playing these and other non-prole games as individuals, as was the case with golf, although their participation was not recorded in *BDN*. However, despite some examples of such traditionally middle-class pursuits such as golf and squash being popular amongst deaf people in some parts of the country, the overall picture is clearly of deaf people having limited involvement in 'non-prole' sports. So whilst deafness does not seem to have acted as a barrier or disincentive in general deaf leisure terms, the same is not true of deaf participation in sports. Why deaf people generally were so outwardly conservative in their sporting enjoyment is not readily apparent, but the range of sports may have been influenced by factors other than merely social class. These might include available facilities, sports first encountered amongst contemporaries in the deaf schools, local tradition, and of course financial restrictions. There is certainly no definitive evidence that conclusively links the range of deaf sports to issues of social class. As with the possible class structure of the deaf clubs, it is not possible to reach any conclusions on this aspect of deaf sport with any degree of certainty.

Indoor sports were a regular feature of the activities of other types of social clubs, so perhaps it should not be surprising that deaf clubs took part in the same sort of activities. They were cheap, relatively easy to organise and opponents were easily found. There is also the advantage that indoor sports are not subject to the vagaries of the weather that can lead to the postponement of outdoors events. Despite the wider range of sports potentially accessible to deaf people, certain factors meant that the scope of organised deaf-centred sport remained restricted. For example, changes in education policy from the 1980s onwards meant that the majority of deaf children were placed in mainstream schools, which meant they often had to travel long distances to school. The provision of shared transport often militated against deaf pupils being involved in any extra-curricular activities, and so access to sport was restricted. The time element of such travel, coupled with a lack of school friends within the local population, were additional factors which reduced opportunities and motivations for deaf pupils to become involved in sporting activity nearer to home. Pupils could also be withdrawn from sport lessons for additional academic lessons, such as improving reading and writing skills. Without an early introduction to various sports, especially outdoor sports, many deaf pupils were lost to sport in later life, or were limited by their lack of skills development. For those pupils who were able to take part in school sports, they were still restricted to those sports that formed part of the school curriculum. Communication with suitable coaches was also an important factor, as without an effective means of explaining rules and tactics, deaf sportsmen and women lacked access to the means to improve or even learn the basics of more technically demanding sports. Whilst the most popular deaf sports might require certain levels of skill, it was also easy to learn the basic elements simply by watching, with no need for complex explanations of rules or tactics. Although deaf sportsmen and women acted as both role models and coaches to younger or less experienced players, they could only do so in sports they themselves had had access to. Deaf sport was certainly less common in the summer than in the autumn and winter months. The shortage of summer sport might suggest a drop in the amount of attendant socialisation, but this was counterbalanced by the number of trips and visits deaf club members made at this time of year. The number of these trips may even have been a contributory factor, as the already comparatively small pool of potential sportsmen and women was further depleted by members choosing to go off on the wide range of holidays and outings outlined above. In this respect, deaf sport can be seen to have been just one part of a much bigger social calendar of events that deaf club members could choose from.

Integration, segregation and notions of disability in deaf sport

In the last quarter of the twentieth century, sport (unlike other leisure activities) was the subject of proactive government initiatives and policies aimed at encouraging integration and interaction between different community groups and responding to the needs of disabled groups in particular. Just how effective these programmes were in promoting sports participation by deaf people is questionable, as they have always shown themselves willing to join in a variety of sporting activities with and against the hearing majority. In terms of activity organised by and through the deaf club, members have been more likely to share sporting contests with hearing people than other leisure activities. This involvement has taken many forms, whether it be through membership of deaf teams, as deaf individuals competing with and against hearing opponents, or as members of teams consisting mostly of hearing players in what might be termed 'hearing sport'. Various sports promotion initiatives have also actively encouraged the greater integration of various minority community groups into the wider community. With the existing network of deaf sporting competitions, and the history of informal integration with hearing sport, deaf sportsmen and women did not need these initiatives, as they already had access to an abundance of sporting opportunities. However, despite this access, deaf sport still fell into a period of decline from the 1990s, suggesting that other factors were responsible.

It is interesting to note that the range of organised deaf sport did not notice-ably expand from the 1970s onwards, when there was a concerted effort to involve a greater number of people in a wider range of sporting activities.[19] Government sponsored programmes such as 'Sport for all' do not seem to have made any significant impact on organised deaf sport in terms of what deaf club members actually took part in. Opportunities for involvement increased for all levels of society from the 1970s onwards, through increased leisure time and the provision of cheap and easily accessible facilities such as leisure centres. Improved access to a range of minority participation or elitist sports meant that deaf people also had access to a number of sports for the first time. Squash was one example of a sport that experienced a huge growth in popularity amongst the general population during the 1970s and 1980s, once access was made easier for a greater number of people. Such increased opportunities meant deaf sportsmen and women were able to broaden their sporting scope on an individual basis, and were no longer as reliant on sport organised solely for deaf competitors. Integration in hearing sport had always been a factor in deaf people's involvement in sport, but now they had access to some sports simply through being able to find sufficient opponents of a suitable standard, through leagues and competitions organised by local leisure centres.

The evidence of the extent of deaf sporting activity most certainly chal-lenges perceptions of deaf people as disabled. De Pauw and Gavron have demonstrated that historically, anyone regarded as being either physically or mentally disabled was thought to be unable to take part fully or 'properly' in either society or, by extension, sport. [20] It is only in recent years that sport amongst disabled groups has been actively promoted for sporting reasons alone. However, Aitchison has shown how the provision of access to sport for disabled people can act as a mechanism for social exclusion, rather than promoting inclusion or integration.[21] The majority of efforts to involve disa-bled people as participants in sport have been based on providing discrete access. This has normally resulted in segregated participation, rather than in promoting access with or alongside 'able-bodied' sportsmen and women. The motivation of those providing access to sports is seemingly based on medical perceptions of disability. There is no apparent acknowledgement of sport as a form of cultural expression for disabled people, despite even segregated sport giving those who take part a sense of shared identity.[22] This attitude should not be surprising, as it is merely an extension of broader assumptions relating to impairment or 'abnormality'. Fullagar and Owler describe how it is the disability that is seen first, and the person second (if at all).[23] This has led to disabled people being excluded from mainstream involvement in leisure and sport through the perpetuation of stereotypes of ability in both disabled and able-bodied groups.

> As a minority (or marginalized) group, individuals with disabilities have limitations placed upon their participation in society. As sport is an integral part of society, similar sanctions and limitations have been imposed for inclusion within the sporting world. [24]

De Pauw and Gavron outline some of the barriers faced by disabled sportsmen, which include a lack of organised sporting events, a lack of role models and psychological and sociological factors.[25] Whilst the economic barrier they identify may have applied to deaf people wishing to become involved in sports, this is not an issue that is unique to deaf or indeed disabled people; many people from all sections of society have faced financial barriers to participation in sport. The evidence contained in the historical record of deaf sport clearly indicates that none of the other factors faced by disabled people, including access to appropriate facilities, have stopped deaf sportsmen and women from regularly taking part in a variety of sports. Older deaf sportsmen and women served as role models and informal coaches, and the only issues of accessibility related to minor alterations in the way in which certain sports were controlled and how the players were notified of the officials' decisions. The fact that other issues, such as the provision of adequate coaching that could meet the communication needs of deaf people, were not widely addressed possibly says more about the attitudes of the sporting bodies than it does about the abilities and potential of deaf sportsmen and women.

Deaf sportsmen and women regularly took part in mainstream sport alongside hearing people, as well as in their own discrete events. The mere presence of deaf sportsmen and women competing alongside their hearing counterparts thus challenges conceptions of both their sporting abilities and wider issues relating to deafness as a disability. This is an often neglected but important aspect of deaf sport. When De Pauw and Gavron assert that 'socialization into sport, let alone socialization via sport, is often not a part of the socialization of youth with disabilities', this does not equate with the experiences of those people who were members of the deaf community.[26] Sport played an important part in their socialisation into a community of people with similar life experiences, backgrounds and expectations. In this respect, deaf sport provided access to a social life that was not generally available to disabled people. When deaf sportsmen and women took part in segregated deaf-only events, this was generally as a matter of choice, sometimes based on social as much as sporting considerations, and was not because of any lack of ability based purely on their being deaf. The sporting history of the deaf community thus acts as an effective rebuttal of claims that deafness should be seen as a disability.

This brief overview of deaf leisure has provided a broad outline of the distribution of deaf clubs across Britain, the types of leisure activities and events deaf club members engaged in as both individuals and collectively, and the ways these changed during the second half of the twentieth century. Whilst there were some minor regional variations and preferences in deaf leisure, these are not sufficiently marked as to warrant detailed examination. The reality is that the evidence presented in *British Deaf News* points to a remarkable and overwhelming similarity of experiences and activity in all parts of the country. Deaf club members in the north of Scotland were taking part in essentially the same types of activities as their counterparts in Kent, Cornwall, Wales and East Anglia. Some activities may have been more popular than others, but in all areas deaf people enjoyed days out and holidays more than any other activity. Everything else came second to this, in even the most remote areas, and deaf people were prepared to go to a great deal of trouble and expense in order to make these journeys – especially when they involved contact with other deaf people. When they did meet, they mixed socially by taking part in similar types of activities wherever that contact occurred.

It is not possible to engage in any large scale analysis on a national level due to the sheer mass of data that *British Deaf News* provides. However, a more detailed unpacking of the realities of deaf leisure is possible on a regional basis and so the next two chapters will provide an examination of the development of leisure practices in north-west England and the way these trends were reflected in deaf club based activities and events during the post-war period. This serves as a case study from which both general and specific aspects of deaf leisure can be identified and discussed, and the principles applied more broadly to other parts of Great Britain. From this analysis, deeper psychological and emotional factors underpinning deaf leisure choices and the way in which these choices have served to support and maintain wider conceptions of community and cohesion amongst deaf people are identified and discussed.

Notes

1   *British Deaf News* (hereafter *BDN*), 1990, p. 15
2   *BDN*, 1975, pp. 108–109
3   *BDN*, 1990, p. 72

4   *BDN*, 1975, pp. 46–47
5   *BDN*, 1990, p. 32
6   For example *BDN*, 1955, p. 88; 1960, p. 13
7   For example *BDN*, 1970, p. 156, p. 220; 1985, September p. 21
8   Examples of these types of activities can be found in *BDN*, 1965, p. 297; 1970, p. 188; 1975, p. 192; 1995, p. 24
9   *BDN*, 1980, p. 234
10   Seguillon, D., 'The origins and consequences of the first World Games for the Deaf: Paris 1924', *The International Journal of the History of Sport* 19, 1 (2003), pp. 119–136
11   Grant, *Deaf advance*; www.britishdeafsportscouncil.org
12   *BDN*, 1980, p. 416
13   Atherton, M., (2007) 'Sport in the British deaf community', *Sport in History* 27, 2: 276–292
14   Atherton *et al.*, *Deaf United*
15   *BDN*, 1985, p. 45
16   Atherton *et al.*, *Deaf United*
17   Atherton *et al.*, *Deaf United*
18   Wilson, T.C., 'The paradox of social class and sports involvement: the roles of cultural and economic capital', *International Review for the Sociology of Sport* 37, 1 (2002), pp. 5–16
19   See Wilson, J., 'Leisure in the welfare state' in C. Critcher P. Brahman and A. Tomlinson (eds), *Sociology of leisure* (London: E & FN Spon, 1995), pp. 216–221; G. Whannel, 'Sport and the state' in Critcher *et al.*, *Sociology of leisure*, pp. 222–228
20   De Pauw, K.P. and S.J. Gavron, *Disability and sport* (Champaign Illinois: Human Kinetics, 1995), p. 9
21   Aitchison, C., 'From leisure and disability to disability leisure: developing data, definitions and discourses', *Disability and Society* 18, 7 (2003), pp. 955–969
22   *Ibid.*
23   Fullagar, S. and K. Owler, 'Narratives of leisure: recreating the self', *Disability and Society* 13, 3 (1998), pp. 441–450
24   De Pauw and Gavron, *Disability and sport*, p. 8
25   *Ibid.*, p. 11
26   De Pauw and Gavron, *Disability and sport*, p. 10

7

LEISURE AND SPORT IN NORTH-WEST ENGLAND SINCE 1945

Case study: Deaf leisure in north-west England

Introduction to this section of the book

The previous chapter provided an overview of the leisure activities of deaf club members across Britain throughout the fifty years from 1945 to 1995. In order to provide a more nuanced examination of deaf leisure in post-war Britain, this study will focus on one part of the country. Whilst no single area can be fully representative of the whole nation, north-west England encompasses many of the different rural and urban environments to be found across Britain. In addition, the number of deaf clubs found across the region and the range of activities their members engaged in provides insights that can be applied to other areas of the country, given the largely homogenous nature of deaf leisure that has already been highlighted.

With this in mind, the next two chapters use this region as a case study of deaf leisure activity across the UK. The first chapter defines the boundaries of north-west England as they apply within this book, and describes the geography and topography for those who are unfamiliar with the region, before moving on to offer a contextualisation of general leisure and sporting activity in the north west during the period of this study. This provides the setting for the following chapter, which investigates the communal and individual leisure pursuits of deaf club members in the region reported in *British Deaf News*. In addition, the chapter demonstrates how deaf people were influenced by the leisure and sporting opportunities available around them and highlights some of the differences between deaf and hearing people's leisure activities. Some of the possible factors influencing deaf club members' choices in spending their spare time are discussed and the somewhat narrow range of sporting activity is analysed, with potential reasons (both identifiable and speculative) for this lack of wider engagement being put forward.

Extensive examples taken from *British Deaf News* are used to provide insights into what deaf people chose to do with their leisure time and how they felt about these activities. These extracts provide a unique insight into the realities of deaf leisure, the importance of such participation in community maintenance and cohesion, and the ways in which deaf club members interacted with the wider hearing population. They also provide evidence of the ways in which such communal leisure first boomed in the 1960s and 1970s before the decline in deaf club membership from the 1980s onwards began to have a serious and adverse effect on shared leisure activities amongst deaf people. The future of deaf leisure and the long term consequences for notions of community and identity engendered amongst deaf people through spending time with others of a similar background are discussed in a national context in the concluding chapter of the book.

Before dealing with the particular aspects of deaf social life in north-west England, it is necessary to set this analysis within the more general context of post-war leisure and sporting activity across north-west England during this period. As a starting point, it is perhaps useful to explain the varied topography and geography of the region and to outline the commercial and industrial infrastructure of north-west England. In order to better understand their leisure choices and practices, this background knowledge allows us to understand what living and working environments the region's inhabitants were taking time off from. Having thus set the scene, this chapter provides a brief history of some of the main elements of social and sporting life in the north west; this in turn helps illustrate the circumstances within which the specific social activities of the area's deaf clubs were located. This examination will concentrate on outlining the communal nature of much of the leisure activity in north-west England, particular that of working-class people, and the ways in which this changed during the period addressed in this study. In doing so, the developments in deaf leisure and sport outlined in the next chapter are given a wider regional context. Certain leisure pursuits have been closely associated with the region and its industrial heritage, and these have contributed to the region's cultural identity. The role of social clubs, particularly in providing and promoting leisure and sport, will be considered, as it is those aspects of deaf life which took place in and around the region's deaf clubs that are of interest.

For the purposes of this study, north-west England is defined as the area extending northwards from the River Mersey to the Scottish border, and eastwards from the Irish Sea coast to the borders with Yorkshire and Derbyshire. These boundaries set the north west within the generally accepted understanding of 'the north' as outlined in Russell's examination of northern identity.[1] In essence, this area consists of the counties of Lancashire, Westmorland and Cumberland as they were constituted prior to county boundary changes in 1974.[2] Those parts of Cheshire that fall within these geographical boundaries, namely Stockport to the south of Manchester, Birkenhead and Wallasey on the Mersey estuary, and Warrington and Widnes, are also included. The map below illustrates the extent of the region and the location of deaf clubs within it.

The region incorporates a wide variety of topography, from the mountainous Lake District to the north, through the moors and valleys of east Lancashire to the wide floodplain of the Mersey to the south. In addition to the Mersey, a number of other major rivers drain the region, including the Irwell, Ribble, Wyre, Lune and Kent. This varied landscape has influenced and been reflected in the economic characteristics of the region throughout the post-war period and in the leisure activities on offer there. The attractions of the Lake District are long established and the coastal plains of west Lancashire and the Fylde in particular have been important centres of leisure activity, as has the vast expanse of Morecambe Bay, with Blackpool, Southport, Fleetwood and Morecambe all having been important holiday destinations.

Agriculture still dominates in the north, particularly hill farming in Cumberland and Westmorland, with industry here restricted largely to the coastal fringes. Other important agricultural areas include west Lancashire between Preston and the coast on both banks of the Ribble.[3] In east and central Lancashire, textile mills comprised the major employer in the immediate post-war years, as they had done since the late eighteenth century. However, textiles experienced a rapid decline from the early 1950s and no longer constituted a significant part of the region's industrial output well before the end of this research but their influence on leisure patterns could still be seen.[4] Coal mining was a major employer throughout the north west, with pits found in the far north west (in the area around Maryport and Workington), east Lancashire (for example in Accrington and Burnley) and across the entire south Lancashire plain. Numerous mines were found in virtually all the towns of this area, such as those around Wigan, Newton-le-Willows, Leigh and St Helens. As with the cotton industry, mining also experienced a gradual and terminal decline from the 1950s onwards as demand from textiles and power stations diminished and geological problems made coal mining increasingly unprofitable. Eighty pits producing over twelve million tons of coal in 1950 declined to only nine active pits by 1975; other than a few opencast mines, there were no working pits left in the north west by 1995.[5]

North-west England

Figure 3 Cities and towns circled indicate the location of deaf clubs
included in this study

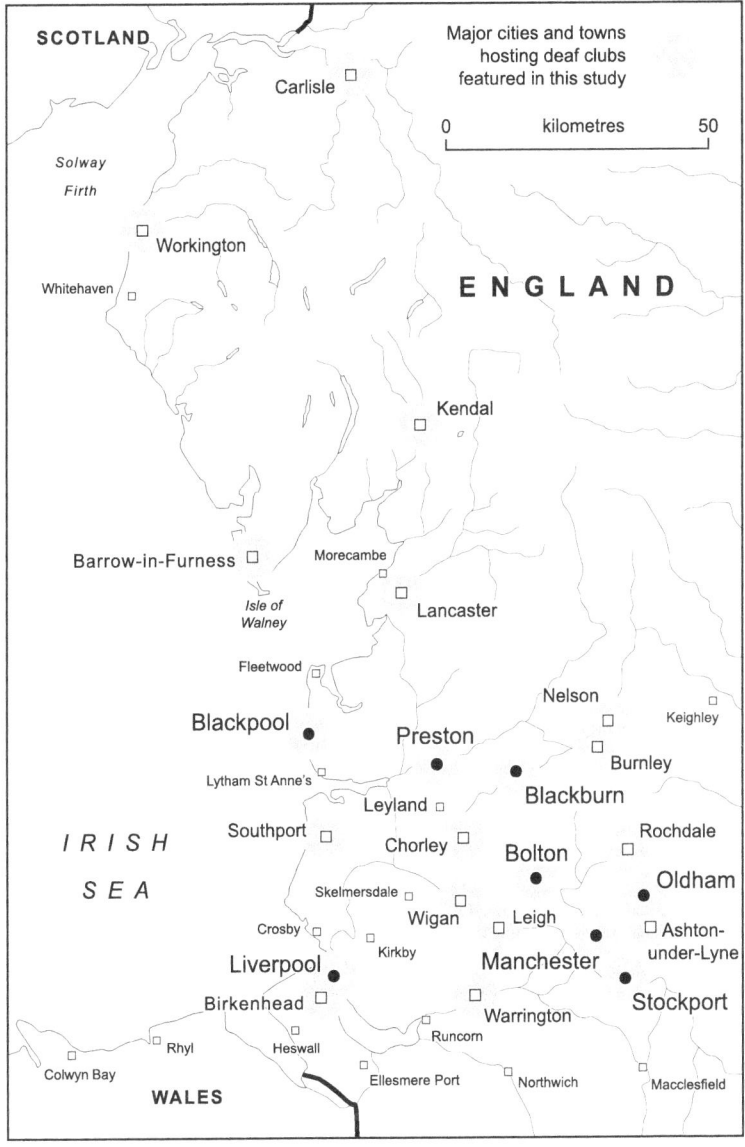

Various other industries were to be found in the region. Shipbuilding took place in Barrow-in-Furness and Birkenhead, imports and exports flowed through the various ports such as Liverpool and Heysham (as well as the inland ports of Manchester and Preston) whilst fishing sustained towns such as Fleetwood and Whitehaven. Glass making was one of the main employers in St Helens, and chemical industries were important contributors to the local economies of towns including Whitehaven, Barrow, Warrington and Widnes. Paper manufacture, serviced by the importing of wood pulp through Preston and Liverpool Docks, was the basis of several large concerns in Blackburn, Warrington and the south Lakes area around Kendal.[6] In addition, both heavy and light engineering concerns were based in many towns; as well as servicing the textile industry, the manufacture of printing presses, trains, cars and commercial vehicles all contributed to the wide range of industries to be found in north-west England.[7] As traditional industries such as textiles and mining declined, new industries such as aircraft manufacture took their place and smaller light engineering concerns and service industries came to be increasingly important as employers. Although the region experienced a severe economic downturn during the 1980s, the diversity of industry allowed sustained economic recovery to occur from the early 1990s.[8] So although cotton is most closely associated with industrial production in the north west, it was by no means the only source of employment or income in the region.

The preponderance of industry, coupled with labour intensive agricultural production, means the majority of the region's population might reasonably be considered to be working class. As Dave Russell has argued, the industrial history of the north west has helped to build a perception of the region amongst outsiders as being to some extent insular, and this has resulted in the inhabitants of the north west being seen to have a strong regional identity, as well as contributing to a broader conception of 'the north' as a whole.[9] This identity has been the subject of much research in relation to leisure and especially sport, in which links between regional and sporting identities can be identified. Several writers have investigated the issue of northern identity from various perspectives, and both the industrial heritage of the region and the leisure activities of its inhabitants – especially the sports enjoyed by the working classes – have been shown to contribute to this commonly held view.[10] This social background, together with other factors such as the proximity of the coast and the types of work people were employed in, all helped to influence the leisure activities enjoyed by the majority of the region's inhabitants. For instance, there are definite links to be found between the textiles towns and the ways in which their inhabitants took their annual holidays, and between specific industries and participation in certain sports. Whilst accepting that the north west was not solely inhabited by working-class people, they did comprise the majority of the population and their activities were more representative of the region's general trends in leisure, sport and culture as a result. Because of this, it is the activities of working-class people from the industrial towns that are paid particular attention here.

Post-war leisure

Following the cessation of hostilities in 1945, the social patterns of the region established before the war began to re-emerge. However, as in many other aspects of post-war regeneration, participation in leisure and sport underwent radical changes during the next fifty years. Established ways of spending free time were supplemented or replaced by new opportunities and aspirations, driven in part by a gradual increase in disposable income and changing attitudes towards leisure as a social activity. As a result, the forms of cultural expression represented by engagement in leisure and sport underwent a period of major change. The cities and towns of the region provided numerous opportunities for their inhabitants to spend their weekly leisure time and disposable income. The prosperity of the region had seen the provision of libraries, art galleries, parks and other civic amenities in towns across the region during the Victorian and Edwardian periods and these were still popular venues for a variety of leisure activities in the years after the Second World War.[11] These sites could assist in the communal expression of the region's cultural heritage, by acting as venues for older local traditions, such as egg rolling. Derived from the older Lancashire tradition of pace-egging, in which boiled eggs were decorated and paraded around parishes and towns, egg rolling still takes place in Preston's Avenham Park every Easter Monday. The townsfolk gather there to roll Easter eggs down the steep slopes of the park, and the continuation of this traditional activity is as closely identified with the setting as it is with the town's communal cultural heritage.[12] For Prestonians, egg rolling was not quite the same when it was performed elsewhere, for example when bad weather meant alternative venues had to be found, such as yards, gardens or even staircases.

A more widely celebrated tradition that gradually disappeared during the post-war period was the Whit Walks. This annual expression of religious and cultural identity manifested itself in the processions of witness that took place in many of the large towns and cities across the north west. Religion had long played an important part in the spiritual and social lives of the region, with the numerous churches also being the organisers of a variety of social and sporting activities for their congregations. The processions served both a religious and a social purpose, with all the churches in a town joining together to march behind their own banners, although there were strict demarcations concerning who marched when. In Preston, the Anglican, Roman Catholic and Free Churches marched on separate days over the extended Whitsun weekend. Great expense was often incurred to fit out participants in new clothes as tradition demanded, whilst attendance at another denomination's procession was often frowned upon.[13] The majority of towns ceased to hold processions of witness from the 1970s, partly due to falling church attendance but also as a spirit of ecumenicalism made such overt displays less acceptable. However, they did continue well into the 1990s in a few places, most notably Liverpool and the hill towns to the east of Manchester, such as Ashton under Lyne and Oldham.[14]

Alcohol and leisure

The consumption of alcohol played a central part in much of the region's leisure life, as it did elsewhere. Each town had an often large number of public houses but there were also a selection of social clubs affiliated to the major political parties or associated with particular trades, sports or interests.[15] These clubs acted as venues for people with common backgrounds, beliefs or interests to meet, socialise and exchange ideas and information. For example, many Catholic churches had their own social clubs, which brought the congregation together in a leisure setting, as well as providing a useful source of supplementary income for the parishes through bar sales. In addition, social clubs served philanthropic purposes such as fundraising for worthy causes and providing care for their members. The various types of social clubs provided support for injured, ill or elderly members, organised group outings to places of interest and holidays and parties for their children. As such, they served as a focus for local community identity. Such clubs went into decline as attendance was replaced by other social habits and although many traditional social clubs still survived towards the end of the twentieth century, their membership had dwindled as younger members were no longer drawn to the clubs in the same numbers as before. The economic impact of the decline in some towns' main employers, particularly the virtual closure of Leyland Motors/British Leyland in Leyland, was another important contributory factor.

However, it would be wrong to claim that the lives of working-class people solely revolved around the regular consumption of alcohol. Indeed, the north west had a long tradition of promoting temperance and abstinence and this was firmly established in the rationale (if not necessarily the working practices) of many working-class leisure and sporting organisations.[16] The first social clubs of this type developed not as drinking establishments but as venues in which members of various trades could take part in a wide range of educational activities. It was on the basis of 'improving' the moral and physical welfare of the working classes that the Club and Institute Union (CIU) was established.[17] The CIU's philosophy was to promote Mechanics Institutes and Working Men's Clubs as alternatives to public houses, as centres of temperance and the providers of rational recreation. It was from these roots that the extensive network of social clubs found in the north west in the years following the Second World War had developed. One factor that did not change was that the most popular activities throughout the period were those which participants took part in communally. As well as informal pursuits based around pubs and social clubs, there were a range of societies and organisations to be found in every town, whilst watching and taking part in a variety of sports was also very popular. As working-class groups took control over their own leisure organisations, many of these clubs and societies continued a tradition of morally or physically improving recreation that had its foundations in the facilities provided by paternalistic employers.

Robert Putnam argues that the decline of society is a result of decreasing voluntary association, and there is certainly evidence of this happening across the north-west as the twentieth century entered its final decades.[18] However it is important to acknowledge that these types of activity did not disappear completely. In some instances, one form of voluntary association was merely replaced by another, although the alternative may have been less formally or rigidly organised. The same changes affected virtually all sections of society across the region, and although the types and venues of these leisure activities changed to some extent, the reasons why people gathered together did not. Whilst forms of leisure that did not involve interaction with other people became increasingly popular, it was still those that involved sharing an activity in the presence of like-minded others that involved the greatest number of participants. Even for popular and apparently solitary activities such as angling or tending allotments, participants often joined clubs and societies associated with these pastimes as they were seeking the same types of psychological rewards that are a major motivating factor in all social activities.

Holidays

The industrial heritage of the region had a major effect on the way many working people from the north west took their most concentrated period of relaxation, their annual holiday. The tradition of Wakes weeks in the Lancashire mill towns dated back well into the nineteenth century and continued into the post-war years; although the term 'Wakes weeks' fell largely into disuse.[19] During the annual holiday period, the majority of factories and associated businesses in the textile towns of the region closed down at the same time, and Blackpool would become Preston-, Blackburn- or Bolton-by-the-sea for a week or fortnight every year as the working populations of these towns would move practically en masse to the Fylde coast. Other Lancashire resorts catered for their own particular clientele, either in terms of their catchment areas or in the type of holiday they provided.[20] Rather than drawing people from Lancashire, Morecambe relied heavily on its rail links with Yorkshire, to the extent that it was known as 'the Yorkshireman's Blackpool', along with a tradition of attracting Scottish visitors for their annual holiday.[21] The more refined Southport, which steadfastly rejected the brasher attractions to be found across the Ribble estuary in Blackpool, provided a genteel day out for the upper- and middle-class inhabitants of Merseyside, with whom it shared an electric train link. Blackpool on the other hand remained the pre-eminent annual destination for workers from across the north west well into the post-war period. Staying in a bed and breakfast hotel, taking donkey rides on the beach, hiring deckchairs on the promenade and watching a show on one of the three piers became a stereotypical view of the Blackpool holiday (largely because this was what a typical holiday in the resort entailed), whilst at the same time being the main reasons why the resort was so popular with its working-class visitors. The resort closely resembled a home from home by the sea in many respects, in addition to offering treats and recreations that were not part of the normal working week. Often, pub regulars, church congregations and social club members would travel as a group, on trips paid for by weekly subs collected (or even paid for) by the pubs and clubs, thus spreading the financial burden over the course of the year.[22] Some employers even continued the earlier practice of providing their workers with free or subsidised holidays.[23]

Eagerly anticipated by the populations of the mill towns, these mass holidays contributed significantly to the continuing popularity of Blackpool in particular after 1945, and despite the growth in overseas holidays and the gradual decline of communal holidays by a town's inhabitants from the early 1970s, this popularity was maintained.[24] John Walton argues that no other industrial area was so closely tied to this type of communal seaside holiday as the industrial north west, and even within the region, areas where other industries dominated did not take their holidays in quite the same concentrated and communal fashion.[25] Nevertheless, these holidays remained closely associated with the region as a whole. Even for those workers from towns that did not close down for a set holiday period, Blackpool was also the primary resort of choice for many years. However, by the 1980s the majority of visitors to the town were making day trips, rather than staying for a week or more as in earlier times, and whole communities no longer holidayed together on such a large scale.[26] Other Lancashire resorts fared less well in the second half of the twentieth century, with Morecambe in particular suffering a major demise as the destination for an extended holiday. Towns such as St Annes and Southport, which had deliberately promoted themselves as suitable destinations for the middle classes, were less seriously affected and also continued to attract day trippers.[27] The phenomenon of the Wakes weeks did not die out completely but from the 1970s onwards it had become the exception rather than the rule for a town to virtually close down for a fortnight whilst its inhabitants went on holiday together, and as a result the social aspects of Wakes weeks gradually disappeared.[28]

Whilst the coastal resorts may have been the most popular holiday destination for working-class people from the north west, these had not been the only type of holiday available to them. Short breaks and holidays in the countryside increased in popularity and day trips for hiking, rambling and fell walking all became important elements in the leisure culture of the inhabitants of north-west towns.[29]

Many of the mill towns had readily accessible countryside nearby, and the proximity of the Lake District and the Yorkshire Dales also catered for those seeking outdoor recreation. The popularity of such activities was assisted by a concerted government policy to promote the countryside as a setting for leisure activities, which led to the creation of the Lake District National Park in 1951.[30] The development of a network of Youth Hostels, which offered basic but cheap overnight accommodation in out of the way places, also contributed to this growth. As the transport network of the region improved in line with the post-war increase in car ownership, a day or weekend of walking on the fells and moors became not only more viable but also more readily available to more people.

As Snape has shown, this built on a long tradition in the north west of taking outdoor exercise dating back well into the nineteenth century and these activities gained in popularity from 1945. This exercise mainly took the form of cycling, rambling and hiking, with the Manchester YMCA Rambling Club, founded in 1880, being just one example of the long history of such well-established organised activity in the north west.[31] These pursuits were promoted as escapes from the often squalid conditions of everyday life in the Victorian towns and holidays in the countryside were organised as alternatives to the perceived immoral temptations to be found in the coastal holiday resorts. The Co-operative Holidays Association (CHA), founded in the east Lancashire town of Colne in 1893, arranged walking holidays in the nearby Yorkshire Dales and attracted members from amongst all classes. The CHA established rambling and fell walking as healthy and morally uplifting activities and took advantage of the extensive areas of lakes, dales and moors within easy travelling distance of all north-west urban areas. The aim of the CHA was not only to provide healthy outdoor holidays, but also to 'promote the intellectual and social interests of its holiday groups'.[32] The tradition of working-class countryside walking was taken up by the British Workers' Sport Federation (BWSF), whose aggressive campaigning for access rights was part of the wider political ambitions of the British Communist Party, of which the BWSF was a social wing. The BWSF's most famous event in the promotion of walking as a working-class leisure activity was the mass trespass on Kinder Scout in the Peak District in 1932. Despite the adverse publicity the action brought to both landowners and the BWSF, the principle of access to the countryside for recreational purposes was established and culminated in the preservation of open spaces as National Parks from 1951.[33]

From the 1960s onwards, overseas holidays began to replace the more traditional seaside holiday at home, with better weather, the novelty of air travel and foreign destinations, and often increased value for money all contributing to the Costa del Sol replacing the Fylde coast in the leisure aspirations of the north west's working-class population. Mediterranean holidays were as cheap as those offered by the traditional Lancashire resorts by the mid-1960s and this hastened the decline of many resorts.[34] This was in line with similar changes taking place across Britain and was helped by the presence of Manchester Airport in the region and the continuing post-war development of airports in Liverpool and Blackpool to meet the growing demand for holiday flights. The combination of a wide range of more appealing overseas destinations within easy reach, more leisure time and disposable income, and a major transport network, meant that travel and outdoor leisure opportunities for those living in the north west increasingly became more varied.

Whilst the large-scale communal nature of annual holidays was broken, groups of friends or club members still travelled together, thus at least partially preserving the tradition of shared holidays that was such a feature of north-west leisure in the years either side of the Second World War. Certain aspects of the leisure lives of people in the north west in 1995 would have been vastly different from those of their earlier contemporaries in 1945, illustrating the way in which many facets of leisure had changed over fifty years. Although many traditional activities continued and indeed flourished in some cases (such as outdoor pursuits), others such as the long-established social clubs appeared to be in serious jeopardy and possibly terminal decline. Whilst leisure remained an important part of the north west's cultural activity, the way in which this culture was expressed and engaged in had undergone a period of extensive change and development.

Sport in north-west England

Similar changes could also be seen in the sporting activities found within the region. Sport, whether engaged in as spectator or participant, had long been an important part of the region's leisure activities, and this continued and indeed increased as working hours shortened (either by design or during periods of industrial decline) throughout the period of this research. As several commentators have shown, sport has played an important role in creating a sense of community identity, and the north west was no different in this respect.[35] Cricket was the most popular sport during the summer months, but it was league cricket rather than the county game that attracted more spectators and was more closely identified with local communities.[36] Clubs represented towns and communities rather than the county as a whole, and local rivalries were much more keenly felt and expressed as a result. This was reflected in the crowds drawn to matches in the Lancashire League, which were measured in their thousands throughout the 1950s and clubs continued to attract significant numbers throughout the third quarter of the century.[37] Each club was allowed (and in some instances required) by league regulations to employ a professional player, and many of the top stars from overseas Test playing countries appeared for town clubs across the region. This led to a high standard of competition and continued a tradition dating back to the 1920s.[38] It was only in the final quarter-century that league cricket began to lose its popularity, as other summer leisure activities become more popular.

Certain sports and pastimes were more closely associated with the region, and in some instances were unique to specific areas. Cumberland and Westmorland wrestling (also known as Cumbrian wrestling), with its unusual attire reminiscent of 'long johns' underwear, was only found in the two counties, where it remains a staple of Lakeland sporting events such as the Grasmere Sports and the Ulverston Games. Whilst these events have historically drawn visitors from beyond the borders of the two counties, they remain uniquely associated with this corner of the north west.[39] Another local activity strongly influenced by the geography of the Lake District is fell running, in which locals race to the top of an overlooking mountain and back. Both these activities acted not only as sporting contests but also served as a means of expressing the cultural identity of the area.[40] Other sports closely associated with the north west could also be found in other regions, but still maintained a close identification with this part of the country. So for example, crown green bowls is often seen as a uniquely north-western game, whilst flat green bowls is perceived as the more widely played version of the sport.[41] However, crown green bowling clubs can be found in the midlands and Wales, whilst flat green bowls was more popular than crown green in certain parts of the north west, especially around Manchester. The first flat green bowling club in the north west was established at Heaton Hall, Stockport in 1926, whilst the Lancashire County Bowling Association was formed in 1951. Crown green bowls has been played for much longer, with inter-county matches dating back to 1893, and with local clubs in existence for many years previously.[42] Both forms of bowls co-existed in the north west throughout the post-war period and served as an important source of sporting competition and social intercourse for their participants during that time. Jeff Hill recounts how another, more esoteric sport closely associated with northern England persisted in east Lancashire until the 1970s. Knur and spell (also known as 'tip and hit' or 'poor man's golf') involved a ball or stone being thrown into the air from a sprung base to be hit with a stick, with the winner being determined by the greatest distance achieved over an agreed number of hits. As late as 1970, a crowd of over 3,000 spectators attended a match in Yorkshire involving the champions of Colne.[43] Although neither could be considered to be uniquely northern pastimes, greyhound and pigeon racing were both popular amongst the region's working class populace. Towns such as Preston and Manchester had dog racing tracks whose meetings were often well attended, whilst pigeon lofts were a common sight in many back yards and gardens. The training of both pigeon and greyhounds was taken very seriously and the rewards to be made from prize money and gambling meant that the results of races were often subject to illegal outside influences.[44] Other forms of racing in the region included speedway, with tracks at Belle Vue in Manchester and Liverpool Stadium, and horse racing. Racecourses in the region included the major tracks at Haydock Park and Aintree in Liverpool, with its national associations with the annual showpiece, the Grand National steeplechase. Smaller tracks could also be found farther north in Carlisle and Cartmel in Cumbria, and all these racing venues provided opportunities for both a sporting day out and the chance to gamble on results through on-course betting.

Professional sport

In the north west, the major forms of mass identification derived through professional sport came from cricket in summer and the major winter games of the region, association football and rugby league.[45] Attendance at a match in either winter sport had been a feature of the leisure activity of the region since the foundation of their respective governing bodies in the late nineteenth century and this continued through the post-war period. The region benefited from the general boom in attendance for all sports in the immediate post-war years, and suffered along with other parts of the country as attendance at foot-ball and rugby slumped during the 1970s and 1980s. The economic conditions in the region were a contributory factor but spectating at professional sports remained an important part of leisure activity in the region, as some indicative attendance figures from the period illustrate. In 1950, there were no less than twenty clubs in the various divisions of the Football League representing the area covered by this study.

The aggregate average attendances of these clubs over the season 1950/51 amounted to 391,910. This figure represents a significant proportion of the region's population attending professional football matches on a regular basis. Whilst it might not be too surprising that a big city club like Everton drew in an average attendance of 42,924, the much smaller town of Preston managed to attract an average of 31,259 fans to every game – figure which represented over 25 per cent of the town's population. Even New Brighton, who suffered from the attraction of their neighbours across the Mersey, managed to draw in an average 4,046 spectators every week.[46] By 1970/71, the nineteen north-west Football League clubs were still attracting 281,403 fans to their matches, including perennial strugglers Barrow and Workington both managing to maintain average crowds in excess of 2,300 and 2,200 respectively.[47] By 1991, two fewer clubs were still drawing 203,718 people through the turnstiles, despite a troubled economic climate.[48] When the crowds of the numerous semi-professional clubs are added – admittedly much smaller than those of the larger Football League clubs but still attracting several hundreds in many cases – then the importance of regularly watching football matches for the inhabit-ants of the region is clear.

Despite regular efforts to expand the geographical base of the game, profes-sional rugby league remains very much a northern sport, with the overwhelm-ing number of clubs to be found in Yorkshire and the north-west of England.[49] Rugby league clubs have always attracted lower attendances than football clubs, due in part to the proximity of many rugby clubs to each other and the comparatively small populations each could draw on compared to football clubs. Research by Tony Collins has shown that average attendances at all Rugby League matches since 1945 have broadly matched that of clubs in the lower tiers of the Football League. Collins found that Rugby League matches in the 1949/50 season drew in almost five million fans, with an average attend-ance across the league of almost 9,500. Although these figures do not indicate levels in the north west, roughly 50 per cent of the clubs were found to the west of the Pennines. Whilst it is not possible to give more accurate figures, a size-able body of people regularly attended Rugby League matches in the region. The decline in Rugby League attendance was even more marked than that in football, and by 1969/70, the total aggregate was down to less than one and a half millions, but recovered slightly by 1989/90 to over 1,600,000.[50] Even allowing for the declining numbers watching both sports from the immediate post-war levels, and taking into account the possibility that some fans would follow both sports, watching the two sports continued to play an important role in the leisure activity of the inhabitants of the north west as the end of the twentieth century approached.

Just as there were distinct patterns to be found in the location of the two types of bowls clubs, so the distribution of football and rugby league clubs also showed some definite geographical distinctiveness. Rugby league clubs were restricted almost exclusively to the areas where coal mining was a major industry or to towns in close proximity to mining areas, which meant they were found mostly in south-west Lancashire and the coastal strip of Cumbria.[51] On the other hand, professional football clubs were found throughout the region, with a total of twenty teams representing virtually every major town and city of the north west in the football league at some point between 1945 and 1995 – except for those in rugby league playing areas.[52] The only towns to boast both professional rugby league teams and clubs in the Football League were Wigan, Blackpool, Barrow and Workington. There were also short-lived teams in the 1980s and 1990s in the football towns of Carlisle and Preston as the Rugby League looked to extend its fan base, but these were introduced into towns with no tradition of supporting rugby league and so did not flourish. This partitioning illustrates the importance of local history and tradition in the continuing popularity of certain sports over others in particular areas. Where no such tradition of spectating exists, as when rugby league clubs were introduced in Preston and Carlisle, the incomers are fighting against established patterns of interest and support in a way that is not found to the same extent in non-sporting leisure activities. These superimposed clubs ultimately failed to attract sufficient support to make them financially viable. This suggests that the attraction of a particular sport as a mass spectator activity has cultural attachments within local communities that are much harder to break down. Although support for individual teams may be somewhat fluid at times and vary according to levels of success, overall support for particular sports is more deeply ingrained. The growth of attendances in football and rugby in recent years also supports this argument, particular in the heartlands of these particular sports that the north west represents.

Participant sports

Sports such as squash, which had previously been of minority interest, were successfully promoted to a wider constituency across the region, particularly from the 1970s onwards. However, none of these new sports managed to establish themselves as major spectator sports; their attraction was mostly for participants. In this, they contributed to the tradition of amateur sport that had a long and extensive history across the north west. The majority of public parks across the region had huge swathes of their grasslands turned over to football and rugby pitches for amateur players and these civic amenities provided venues for cricket and bowls clubs in summer, in addition to the number of private clubs offering sporting facilities. Some indication of the opportunities available – whether as player, official, administrator or spectator – is provided by an examination of amateur sport in Preston. Various sporting bodies and organisations in the town reported their results and competitions in the pages of the local newspaper, the *Lancashire Evening Post*. Although the coverage varied over the years and was by no means exhaustive, it is possible to gain insights into at least some of the amateur sporting life of the town. Based on the last full week in April, when there was an overlap of winter and summer sports, the same years were investigated as those used for assessing attendance at professional sport. In 1951, football clubs from Preston could be found playing in the West Lancashire League, the Lancashire Amateur League and the Lancashire Combination. Within the town, amateur footballers could choose from the Preston and District League, the Preston Churches League and the Preston and District Catholic League, all of which had several divisions and numerous clubs. The town's half-day closing gave rise to midweek afternoon football in the Preston Thursday League, which included teams representing a number of local companies as well as sides from the local army barracks.

During the summer months, football gradually gave way to cricket and bowls. Preston Cricket Club were members of the semi-professional Northern League and the Palace Shield competition included several local clubs from the town. The town was also represented by clubs in other amateur leagues including the Lancashire League and the Ribblesdale League. Crown green bowlers could take part in the Preston and District Bowling League whilst Labour clubs had their own Federated League, both of which involved multi-player teams playing in several divisions. Many other sports were also locally available, including boys' and men's boxing clubs, snooker leagues, tennis in several private clubs and on public courts and rugby union at Preston Grasshoppers. Preston Harriers provided athletics, there were two cycling clubs and Preston also boasted a greyhound track at which many local trainers raced their dogs. Indoor activities included various darts and snooker competitions, and the local baths hosted several swimming galas. Many more opportunities were available within easy travelling distance, such as a table tennis exhibition tournament in Bolton.[53] These various leagues had been both expanded and augmented by the emergence of other leagues by 1971. The Lancashire Evening Post Sunday League included forty-eight teams whilst the Churches League and Catholic League had well over fifty teams between them. When those playing in the other football leagues are added, it is clear that amateur football was providing exercise and sporting opportunities for a great many of the town's men. A similar situation could be found in the summer months, with the Palace Shield involving at least two teams from each of twenty cricket clubs, in addition to the parks-based Churches and Catholic Leagues. One bowls league alone involved ninety-eight teams, each of which numbered seven players.

Indoor sports were equally popular, with the Preston and District Table Tennis League featuring forty-two teams spread across three divisions.[54] Local amateur sport was not reported as extensively in 1991, but the continuing popularity and importance of some sports can still be gauged. There were ten different bowling leagues in the Preston area, involving 482 teams in forty-six different divisions. The Preston and District League alone had fifteen divisions of ten teams each. This represents a huge number of people, even allowing for the likelihood that a proportion of bowlers were playing for several clubs in different competitions. Ten pin bowling also appeared in the newspaper in 1991, the five division competition of forty-five teams indicating the popularity of the sport's revival at the time. The table tennis league in Preston doubled in size from 1971 and now featured eighty-four teams.[55] These levels of activity are by no means all that was taking place in Preston in these years, but they do serve to show just how many people were involved in sport in some form. This involvement would be replicated proportionately in virtually every town across the north west, and gives some indication of the numbers involved in amateur sport. As well as taking part in these sports, strenuous efforts were also put into organising training, fundraising and social events based around the football, rugby, cricket or bowls club. Because of the diversity and extent of involvement in local amateur sports, the impact of sport was felt far beyond those who actually took to the field of play. For example, cutting and marking out the large number of football and cricket pitches was a major task and the number of football kits alone that needed washing every winter weekend required a large support network – whether willing or otherwise.

Sport in the north west was not merely restricted to those sports outlined above. Horse racing, golf, tennis, swimming, athletics and a range of other outdoor sports such as rugby union and lacrosse could all be found within the region in the post-war period. However, other than attending race meetings, many of these sports were often the preserve of the middle classes and as a result never gained the same hold on the majority of the region's population.[56] Indoor activities based in the working-class pubs and clubs also flourished, with leagues for snooker and billiards (and latterly pool), darts, and various types of competitive card games to be found in every town. As government initiatives such as 'Sport for all' sought to involve greater numbers of people in a wider range of sporting activities, so public and private leisure facilities increased. Leisure centres appeared in every major conurbation; in some towns such as Preston and Blackburn, more than one such facility was built. Previously minority or elitist sports such as squash and golf benefited from greater numbers of participants as access was improved, fees and equipment became cheaper and coaching became more widely available. Some longer established sports declined, as leisure habits and fashions changed, with league cricket being a prime example. Attendances had dwindled from crowds in their thousands in the 1950s to often little more than a few dozen by the 1990s, whilst fans returned in their droves to the football grounds of the region. The fact that so many people rediscovered their attraction to these (and other) sports – for whatever reason - illustrates their continuing importance in the social and cultural life of the north west.

Changes in leisure participation

Leisure and sport in north-west England underwent a series of major changes between 1945 and 1995. This was not the result of any inadequacy in the range of leisure and sporting opportunities available across the region; indeed the opposite was true. The changes that occurred were instead indicative of the changes occurring in society generally during this period. In leisure pursuits, people no longer identified or associated with others based primarily on shared employment or residence to the extent they had in 1945. The opportunities for acquiring sporting identity increased, and whilst people remained attached to particular teams, clubs and sports, local ties became less important in attracting people to these activities. Improved transport and increased disposable income, combined with a changing social climate that often valued success more than locality, meant that loyalties became more fluid. As participation in sports also became less restricted to what was available locally and choice increased, so patterns of involvement changed. The social and sporting life of the north west in 1995 was significantly different in many aspects from that of 1945, despite the constancy of some elements. What people did in their free time might not necessarily have changed in terms of watching or playing sport, going on holiday, or enjoying the company of others. However, various elements of leisure activity and social life most certainly had, particularly for the majority of the region's population – its working class. The range of activities they had the opportunity to take part in expanded; the venues for these leisure activities were different from those to which their parents had access, such as their holiday destinations or the venues in which they gathered together socially; whom they shared their leisure time with also changed, as ties of community through common residence or occupation weakened. How – or indeed if – these broader changes were reflected in the social lives of deaf people living in north-west England will be considered in the next chapter.

Notes

1   Russell, D., *Looking north: northern England and the national imagination* (Manchester: Manchester University Press, 2004), pp. 14–18

2   Cumbria was created in 1974 from the merger of Westmorland and Cumberland, together with parts of Lancashire

3   Chaloner, W.H., *Palatinate studies: chapters in the social and industrial history of Lancashire* (Manchester: Carnegie, 1992) and W. Rollinson, *A history of Cumberland and Westmorland* (Chichester: Phillimore, 1996)

4   Singleton, J., 'The decline of the British cotton industry since 1940' in M.B. Rose (ed.), *The Lancashire cotton industry: a history since 1700* (Preston: Lancashire County Books, 1996), pp. 296–324; L.G. Sandberg, *Lancashire in decline: a study in entrepreneurship, technology and international trade* (Columbus: Ohio State University Press, 1974)

5   Crosby, A., *History of Lancashire* (Darwen: Phillimore, 1998), pp. 118–119; C.B. Phillips and J.H. Smith, *Lancashire and Cheshire from AD 1540* (London: Longman, 1994), pp. 327–330

6   Phillips and Smith, *Lancashire and Cheshire*, pp. 317–320

7   Clark, T., *A century of shipbuilding: products of Barrow in Furness* (Lancaster: Dalesman, 1971); Crosby, *History of Lancashire*; D. Hay, *Whitehaven: an illustrated history* (Beckermet: Michael Moon, 1979); Hunt, *Preston*; P. Marlow, *Liverpool: looking out to sea* (London: Cape, 1993)

8   Crosby, *History of Lancashire*, pp. 118–119

9   Russell, *Looking North*

10 See Collins, T., *Rugby's great split: class, culture and the origins of Rugby League football* (London: Frank Cass, 1998); Hill and Williams, *Sport and identity*; M. Huggins, 'The regular re-invention of sporting tradition and identity: Cumberland and Westmorland wrestling c. 1800–2001' *The Sports Historian* 21, 1 (2001), pp. 35–55

11 Hunt, *Preston*, pp. 214–217 and Kidd, *Manchester*, pp. 156–164 offer descriptions of typical civic provision of leisure and recreation facilities in the north west

12 Crosby, A., *The Lancashire dictionary of dialect, tradition and folklore* (Otley: Smith Settle, 2000), pp. 75, 149

13 Crosby, *The Lancashire dictionary*, pp. 211–213

14 Kidd, *Manchester*, pp. 120–122

15   Hill, J., *Sport, leisure and culture in twentieth century Britain* (Basingstoke: Palgrave, 2002), pp. 130–145

16   Levitt, I., *Joseph Livesey of Preston: business, temperance and moral reform* (Preston: University of Central Lancashire, 1996). See also G.P. Williams and G.T. Brake, *Drink in Great Britain 1900 to 1979* (London: Edsall, 1980) and Hunt, *Preston*, pp. 198–204

17   The philosophy of the founders of Working Men's Clubs and the aims of the Club and Institute Union are outlined at www.infed.org/thinkers/solly

18   Puttnam, *Bowling alone*

19   Hudson, J., *Wakes week* (Stroud: Alan Sutton, 1992)

20   Walton, J.K., *Wonderland by the waves: a history of the seaside resorts of Lancashire* (Preston: Lancashire County Books, 1992); J.K. Walton, *The Blackpool landlady: a social history* (Manchester: Manchester University Press, 1978)

21   Fowler, A., *Lancashire cotton operatives and work, 1900–1950* (Aldershot: Ashgate, 2003), p. 63

22   *Ibid.*, pp. 63–64; Walton, *Wonderland*, pp. 18–19

23   Walton, *Wonderland*, p. 16

24   Walton, *Blackpool*, pp. 138–161

25   *Ibid.*, p. 21

26   Crosby, *History of Lancashire*, pp. 142–147

27   Walton, *Wonderland*, pp. 37–39

28   Crosby, *History of Lancashire*, pp. 142–147

29   Smith, P., *Lancashire speaks* (Lancaster: Carnegie Publishing, 1999), pp. 126–138

30   Snape, R., 'The Co-operative Holidays Association and the cultural formation of countryside leisure practice' *Leisure Studies* 23, 2 (2004), pp. 143–158

31   *Ibid.*, p. 144

32   *Ibid.*, p. 146

33   Phillips and Smith, *Lancashire and Cheshire*, pp, 352–354

34   Crosby, *History of Lancashire*, p. 143

35   See Bradley, J.M., 'The patriot game' *International Review for the Sociology of Sport* 37, 2 (2002) pp. 17–197; R. Holt, 'Heroes of the north: sport and the shaping of regional identity' in Hill and Williams, *Sport and identity*, pp. 137–164; J. MacClancy (ed.), *Sport, identity and ethnicity* (Oxford: Berg, 1996)

36   Holt, 'Heroes of the north', pp. 144–150

37   Fowler, *Lancashire cotton operatives*, pp. 66–69

38   Hill, *Nelson*, p. 119–126

39   See Barnes, F., *Barrow and district* (Barrow: Barrow in Furness Corporation, 1968), p. 125

40   Huggins, 'Cumberland and Westmorland wrestling' provides an analysis of wrestling in the social and cultural identity of the Lake District counties

41   Holt, *Sport and the British*, pp. 156–159

42   British Crown Green Bowls Association (www.bowls); Lancashire County Bowling Association (www.lineone.net/~lancsba/county_his.htm)

43 Hill, *Nelson*, pp. 116–117

44 Holt, *Sport and the British*, pp. 185–189

45 Holt, 'Heroes of the north' , p. 138

46 Tabner, B., *Through the turnstiles* (Harefield: Yore Publications, 1992), p. 98

47 *Ibid.*, p. 118

48 *Ibid.*, p. 138

49 Holt, 'Heroes of the north', pp. 157–160

50 Collins, T., *Rugby League in twentieth century Britain* (London: Routledge, 2006)

51 Russell, D., ' "Sporadic and curious": the emergence of rugby and soccer zones in Yorkshire and Lancashire, 1850–1914', *International Journal of the History of Sport* 5, 2 (1988), pp. 185–205

52 Nawrat, C. and S. Hutchings, *The Sunday Times Illustrated History of Football* (London: Hamlyn, 1997)

53 Details drawn from issues of the *Lancashire Evening Post* (*LEP*), 21 to 27 April 1951

54 *LEP*, 23 to 29 April 1971

55 *LEP*, 22 to 28 April 1991

56 Holt, R., 'Heroes of the north', p. 160

8

THE LEISURE LIVES OF DEAF PEOPLE IN NORTH-WEST ENGLAND, 1945–1995

The range of activities constituting deaf leisure in post-war Britain is worthy of closer examination. This chapter will therefore analyse the activities of the 28 deaf clubs in north-west England as they were reported in *British Deaf News*. The social lives of deaf club members will be discussed in terms of their general leisure activities and by their involvement in a variety of sports. Because of the similarity of deaf leisure across the UK, factors such as choice and preference, motivation and opportunity, together with the emotional and psychological rewards of leisure and sport participation can all be investigated in the context of north-west England and the findings applied more broadly to deaf leisure nationally.

The scope of deaf leisure

The 'Around the Clubs' pages of *British Deaf News* illustrate both the breadth and depth of deaf leisure across north-west England, with 1,642 separate leisure events reported and a further 573 relating to sporting involvement. When broken down into the eleven broad categories previously identified, the popularity of each can be assessed:

Table 4 The popularity of leisure activities of deaf club members

Dances and parties (16%)	Fundraising events (15%)
Anniversaries and presentations (8%)	Church and religious events (12%)
Societies and courses (4%)	Community events (4%)
Practical demonstrations and talks (5%)	Trips and holidays (24%)
OAP events (5%)	Youth and children events (2%)
Cards (2%)	

Of the 1,643 events reported, 402 were trips, visits or holidays, representing 24 per cent of the total number of events reported. Attendance at dances (usually referred to as dinner dances) and parties constituted the second most popular activity, with 16 per cent of deaf club social life being devoted to this type of event. Fundraising was the third most reported deaf club activity, at 15 per cent; given the way in which most deaf clubs had to fund and support themselves, perhaps it should not be too surprising to learn that holding social events to raise funds accounted for a significant proportion of the members' efforts. The continuing influence of church and religious groups in deaf life is shown by the number and regularity of reports on church based events, although these show a marked decline towards the end of the century.

There was no activity missing that one might expect to find in the leisure activities of members of similar types of social clubs, although the lack of reports on bingo, which was one of the weekly features of deaf club life, might seem problematic. However, bingo was as commonplace in the clubs as drinking and chatting and so perhaps it was considered too mundane to report in *BDN*. Another activity which members regularly and consistently engaged in was playing card games. Unlike bingo, there were regular reports of cards games, which served a competitive purpose through clubs' involvement in various in indoor sports leagues. In addition, whist drives and the like were also arranged as informal social events within the deaf clubs. Because of this internal social aspect, playing cards is included under the heading of leisure activities rather than sport.

Trends in the popularity of activities

Although there are some fluctuations in the level of activity reported during the research period, the overall trend was one of increasing involvement in communal leisure activity until 1970 (rising from 21 reported events in 1945 to 231 in 1970). Factors such as greater disposable income and more leisure time for deaf club members may account for at least some of the increase. This would also correlate with the trend of greater leisure activity amongst the general population during the same period. Following a period of decline during the 1980s, when Britain experienced a period of economic depression, there was a further rise in deaf club-based leisure activity until 1995 (263 recorded events), since when membership of deaf clubs across the UK has gone into serious – and in all likelihood terminal – decline. So in many ways, the period 1945 to 1995 might be seen as the golden age of deaf clubs and deaf communal leisure.

As well as differences in the number of activities, there were also specific geographical differences in the type of activities enjoyed across north-west

England. For example, Blackburn was by far the most active club in terms of forging links with the wider community through shared leisure and social activity. The club accounted for 22 per cent of all such events, and members were involved in a range of activities with local hearing people and groups. Cumbria's deaf clubs have a longer history of involvement within the wider community than other areas, which may be partly due to the British Deaf Association's headquarters being based in Carlisle until the late 1980s. This may well have given deaf people a higher than usual profile amongst the local hearing population, leading to increased incidences of cross-community engagement and interaction. The comparative isolation of the clubs in Cumbria may have been another factor, forcing deaf clubs to compensate for the difficulties of meeting other deaf groups by having greater involvement with hearing groups. However, deaf leisure was far from restricted to purely local activities, with deaf people regularly seeking (and taking) opportunities to socialise outside of their own area. Although not a great deal of activity was reported in some years by deaf clubs in Wigan or Bolton for example, deaf people from these towns travelled to the busier deaf clubs in Manchester to join in with their events instead. This fluidity of communal leisure is one of the distinguishing features of deaf club life and helps to explain the sheer number of trips deaf club members made. Deaf people's enjoyment of visits to and by other deaf people provides an insight into the wider leisure motivations of deaf people, and serves to emphasise the culturally defining nature of many deaf club-based activities.

Visits and trips

Making trips and visits together was by far the most popular group activity for deaf club members, representing a quarter of all reported activities by north-west deaf clubs, a figure that remained fairly constant throughout the period of this study. This heading includes visits and trips organised under the auspices of individual deaf clubs to a wide variety of venues and events, as well as communal holidays taken by club members.

The majority of these reports refer to organised trips made by groups of north-west deaf club members, although there were also numerous reports of deaf club members from other parts of the country – and beyond – paying visits to deaf clubs in the region. Lancaster Deaf Club hosting a party of forty-five members from Nottingham Deaf Club in 1950, and Wigan making a similar trip to visit Sheffield Deaf Club are just two examples of the post-war revival in this aspect of deaf life.[1] When a party from West London Deaf Club travelled up to Liverpool in 1950, their counterparts from Liverpool Deaf Club showed them around the city and provided entertainment in the evening before the

Londoners returned home.[2] From 1955 onwards, making and hosting visits and trips became the most popular activity amongst north-west deaf club members. Examples of visitors being greeted in north-west deaf clubs were found throughout the post-war period, with Warrington hosting Bradford Deaf Club in 1960 and Carlisle welcoming York Deaf Club in 1970.[3] In 1980, Barrow Deaf Club reported the annual visit of Bedford Deaf Club to Cumbria, during which the southern members joined their northern hosts in a number of trips around the Lake District and enjoyed specially arranged social events.[4] These types of 'incoming' reports are perhaps unsurprisingly most prevalent in reports from Blackpool Deaf Club, which opened its doors to the regular parties of deaf visitors who chose to take holidays in the town. Long distance visitors to the resort included groups from both Gillingham and Southampton Deaf Clubs in 1990, and Aberdeen Deaf Club's earlier trip to view the illuminations in late 1965 was just one of a number of similar visits which invariably included a social event at the town's deaf club.[5] Whilst Blackpool Deaf Club provided deaf visitors to the resort with a social retreat in the evenings, an additional burden was placed upon the members. Many casual visitors seem to have expected Blackpool Deaf Club to organise accommodation on their behalf once they arrived in the town. The problem was apparently so acute in the 1950s that Blackpool Deaf Club was forced to place a notice in *British Deaf News* asking visitors not to expect this service in the future.

Special Notice

Owing to the number of people who came to Blackpool without booking accommodation, and for whom quite a lot of time was spent looking for same, some late at night, notice is now given that we cannot accept responsibility for finding accommodation for those who come here during the two weeks preceding the August Bank Holiday weekend and the two weeks after.[6]

It appears that deaf hospitality has its limits, whatever the strengths of the deaf community.

Many of these trips were for a comparatively short time, despite often travelling quite long distances. Middlesbrough's visit to Liverpool in 1985 and Stoke Deaf Club travelling to Kendal in 1995 were typical day trips, although improved road connections admittedly made such trips less arduous than in earlier years.[7] All these trips were in addition to the numerous instances of north-west clubs visiting their near-neighbours for a range of social and sporting events, often combining the two. Some trips into the area had an international flavour, as deaf visitors from abroad sought out north-west deaf clubs for informal cultural and social exchanges. Such exchanges included German visitors visiting both Whitehaven and Barrow Deaf Clubs during their tour around the Lake District in 1985, Irish and Canadian visitors calling at Carlisle in 1990, and a deaf group from Malta visiting Stockport Deaf Club in the same year.[8] Deaf visitors from the Gambia were to be found in Merseyside in 1995.[9] It is a common misconception that there is only one form of sign language, which is the same no matter what the country of origin of the deaf person, but there are in fact a number of different and distinct sign languages to be found around the world. However, a lack of knowledge of other languages poses less of a problem for sign language users than it does for those who use speech. It is much easier for sign language users to adapt to different varieties of sign languages, due to the visual nature of the language, and a shared *lingua franca* can be fairly easily established, making communication much more easily achievable than it might be for two groups of hearing people, whose languages may be mutually unintelligible.[10]

Such international exchange visits were reciprocated, with organised club trips ranging far and wide across Europe from the 1960s onwards. These were in addition to the trips made by small groups of members travelling independently. As early as 1955, a Barrow Deaf Club member visited Belgium and France, calling at a number of deaf clubs in the towns he visited.[11] In the same year, Liverpool Deaf Club reported that one of its members was 'by now a seasoned foreign traveller' who travelled to Denmark for a sporting tournament, whilst other members spent holidays in Austria, Switzerland, France and Yugoslavia.[12] In 1970 a group from Preston Deaf Club visited Innsbruck in Austria, during which time they paid a prearranged visit to the town's deaf club for the obligatory social evening.[13] Liverpool Deaf Club organised a visit to Ghent Deaf Club in Belgium five years later, as part of an Easter trip to take part in a football tournament; this combination of sporting and social events was a regular part of the activities of deaf clubs, with Manchester Deaf Football Club's trip to Germany in 1985 being another such multi-purpose trip.[14]

Deaf club outings could also have a broader cultural or educational purpose, with trips to the theatre and cinema, or to museums and gardens becoming increasingly common from the 1960s onwards. Southport Deaf Club members visited the stately home at Alton Towers in 1970, in its pre-adventure park days, as did Stockport Deaf Club in 1975, whilst Southport went on a mystery tour to Whalley Abbey in the Ribble Valley.[15] In 1985, Blackpool Deaf Club paid visits to both Castle Howard and the National Garden Festival. Bolton Deaf Club also chose this latter destination for a day trip.[16] Beamish Open Air Museum in County Durham was the joint destination of Carlisle and Pendle Deaf Clubs in 1990, with the trip coinciding with the filming of an item for BBC TV's *See Hear* programme for deaf viewers.[17] Educational trips included

Wigan members visiting a local power station in 1960 to learn how electricity was generated, which was followed by a visit to the Wedgwood pottery factory in 1965; 1970 saw Warrington Deaf Club visiting a motor museum and Bolton members were invited to their local Fire Brigade headquarters, whilst Blackpool Deaf Club's trips in 1995 included visits to Pilkington Glass Works, Appleby Horse Fair and the Ironbridge Gorge.[18] These are just a few examples of what were literally hundreds of such trips, which increased in popularity from the 1960s to the 1980s, despite the growth of the more exotic trips abroad. The variety and regularity of these outings shows that deaf people were not insular when making leisure choices, and nor did they restrict themselves merely to deaf-oriented activities.

Not all international trips made by deaf club members included or required interaction with the local deaf community in the countries visited. As foreign holidays became a more regular part of the leisure activities of Britons generally during the 1960s and 1970s, similar trends can be found in the north-west deaf community. News of overseas holidays – either by members travelling independently, or as organised deaf club trips – became a regular feature of the 'Around the Clubs' pages of *BDN* from the 1960s onwards. Deaf club members from Wigan arranged camping holidays in France, a sea cruise and a group holiday in the south of France in 1960, when such trips were not yet as commonplace amongst the general population as they became later in the decade.[19] Five years later, Wigan members were to be found holidaying in Italy and Spain, whilst in the same year, eleven members of Oldham Deaf Club travelled together on a package holiday to Majorca.[20] The 1970s explosion in overseas holidays, particularly to destinations where sunshine was guaranteed, did not pass deaf club members by, with Blackpool members taking a group holiday in Benidorm in 1975, a holiday which twenty-two members of the same deaf club repeated in 1980.[21] In 1975 Liverpool members visited Austria as part of a gathering of deaf club members from across the country; Preston Deaf Club members, having visited Innsbruck in 1970, were reported to be planning a trip to Sweden for the following year and chose Holland as their destination in 1975.[22] The same year saw the club embark on a much more ambitious project, as 120 members went on a cruise of the Mediterranean and the Canary Islands.[23] The cruise must have been a huge undertaking to organise, and serves as an extreme but by no means remarkable example of the way in which the community life of a deaf club extends beyond the physical boundaries of the building in which the deaf club is held. In effect, the cruise ship became the *de facto* deaf club for the duration of the holiday.

Two Pendle members stretched the boundaries of such holidays further when they organised a group trip to Bulgaria in 1990, and the holiday aspirations of deaf people in north-west England were reflected in their personal holiday choices, which included the Canaries, the US, Malta and Corfu.[24] Two Pendle members celebrated their Silver Wedding anniversary with a cruise in the Mediterranean on which they were accompanied by other members of Burnley Deaf Club; the same club also arranged a caravanning holiday in Spain for its members.[25] The growth in holiday destinations generally was also demonstrated by the selection of the Caribbean, Switzerland, Gibraltar, the West Indies, Egypt, Zambia and Hawaii by members of various deaf clubs across the north west.[26] This breadth of choice for holidays and the number of such holidays being taken shows that far from being isolated and in need of care and support, many deaf club members found no financial or logistical difficulties in emulating their hearing neighbours when it came to choosing and taking holidays.

The 'deaf holiday'

The way in which a deaf club outing regularly incorporated a visit to another deaf club may be seen as being a culturally defining aspect of deaf social life. Whilst other social groups may have occasionally come together for shared events (for example, the Yorkshire and Durham Miners Galas to which Miners Welfare Clubs organised outings), no other network of social clubs seems to have such an extensive history of collective leisure events as deaf club members. The question of why deaf people have chosen to do so remains to be addressed; the example of what might be termed 'deaf holidays' may provide an answer.

One type of trip that was extremely popular in both the number of reports and the value placed upon it by deaf people was the communal holiday, and there are numerous reports of such trips to be found in the pages of *BDN*. In many respects these were often merely longer versions of the regular day trips all clubs made. Communal holidays tended to fall into two main categories: the group holiday organised by and for members to a variety of destinations (as discussed above); and the centrally organised holidays in which members of a number of deaf clubs would gather together in one location, often taking over a holiday camp or similar venue for a week or fortnight. From 1955 onwards, these were annual events for most clubs, with certain clubs choosing to visit the same resorts year on year. Many of these types of communal holidays were often paid for from club funds and provided free of charge, particularly when those being catered for were pensioners or disadvantaged in some way. Blackpool Deaf Club reported in 1960 that their OAP members would once again be making their annual journey to Southport for a week's break.[27] By 1970, the venue had changed to Scotland and the fifty-five Blackpool members on the holiday were said to include a number of 'infirm' members.[28] Liverpool Deaf Club paid for their deaf-blind members to have a week's holiday in Blackpool in 1955, and Wigan Deaf Club organised a similar holiday to Scarborough for their deaf-blind members in 1960.[29]

Many deaf clubs arranged annual holidays in resorts such as Blackpool, and the dates of these were co-ordinated to ensure that several deaf clubs were present in the same town at the same time. These communal holidays mirrored the region's Wakes weeks tradition, and indeed continued long after such shared relaxation had largely been abandoned by the non-deaf residents of the north west. Wigan, Bolton and Southport Deaf Clubs' joint holiday in Paignton in 1965 is just one example, and the annual Blackpool Rally saw literally hundreds of deaf people of all ages descend on the resort for an extended weekend. By 1990, the Rally had evolved into an event aimed primarily at young adults and attracted over 500 younger deaf people to the resort that year.[30] Another important social gathering was the annual BDA Conference, which although concerned with campaigning on deaf issues, was also incorporated in the holiday plans of many delegates. Whether the seaside venues for the conference were chosen to attract more people to attend the conference is not clear, but nevertheless the conference was as much a social and cultural gathering as it was a political event.

The British Deaf Association organised their own series of members' holidays, particularly during the 1960s to 1980s, and these were popular because they brought together deaf people from around the country. In many respects, the BDA was replicating the work of organisations such as the Co-operative Workers Association and the Workers Travel Association in providing group holidays for their members.[31] Where the BDA differed slightly was in not having their own discrete facilities; instead deaf people took over a hotel or holiday camp for the duration of the event. Even as recently as 1995 (the last year covered by this research), Burnley and Liverpool Deaf Clubs were amongst those taking part in the BDA holiday in Scarborough.[32] In 1990 the BDA Centenary Rally was held in Brighton, and members of several north-west deaf clubs took advantage of the long weekend break to join in the festivities.[33] Travelling comparatively long distances to be involved in BDA holidays does not seem to have deterred north-west deaf club members, as both Blackburn and Southport Deaf Clubs travelled to Bournemouth in 1965 and various deaf clubs from across Manchester descended on Lowestoft and Skegness in 1975.[34] The Isle of Wight and the Isle of Man were other popular and regular destinations for BDA holidays attended by north-west members. Particular interest groups were also catered for, with members from Pendle amongst those taking part in Deaf Camping and Caravanning Club gatherings during the 1980s and 1990s.[35] Manchester Deaf Club attended the 1965 Deaf Motorists Rally in Scarborough, whilst Lancaster and Warrington Deaf Clubs were amongst several clubs at the event in 1970, during which Warrington won the 'Motoring Quiz' and the national Road Safety Competition organised by the British Deaf Association.[36] Thus even holidays could be utilised for educational purposes and the spirit of 'rational recreation' lived on in certain aspects of deaf leisure.

By bringing deaf people together on these holidays, variety was introduced into deaf social life, as those taking part had the opportunity to meet new friends and renew existing acquaintances. This was particularly important before the introduction of technology such as the textphone, which now allows deaf people to communicate easily and quickly with each other via the telephone system. Prior to these devices being available, deaf people had no way of maintaining direct contact with other deaf people except by letter or via face to face communication. One of the attractions of the deaf club was that it provided an opportunity for deaf people to meet and socialise that was not available in other elements of their lives. Shared holidays therefore served as a temporary extension of the members' own deaf club, with a greatly enhanced membership brought together for a longer period of time unencumbered by the demands of everyday life. Visits to other deaf clubs served a similar purpose over a shorter period. In effect, deaf people gathering together for a shared activity might be seen to derive additional benefits to those normally associated with holidays specifically and leisure activities generally. Holidays provide an escape from the pressures of everyday life and the chance to engage in 'abnormal' (i.e. non-routine) activities. The same is of course true of deaf people, but when they gather together, they are in fact escaping from a daily experience that is in some respects abnormal.

Deaf sign language users do not usually have the same opportunities to engage in the type of social intercourse that is an integral and important part of working with other people. Just as with membership of a deaf club, sharing holidays and other leisure activities with those from a similar background offered deaf people the chance to share in a more fulfilling way of life for at least part of the year. This allowed the sociological and psychological benefits that accrue from membership of a deaf club to be experienced beyond the physical confines of the deaf club's base. Thus the term 'deaf club' is not restricted to a fixed physical space but can also be considered to mean a group of people choosing to associate with each other. This point will be returned to later in the final chapter, when the issues of topophilia and 'home' will be addressed in the context of deaf clubs.

Not all deaf club members could take part in the trips organised by their clubs, but those left behind could still share in the experience to some degree. Many clubs had keen cine-photographers amongst their members and they regularly recorded club trips and showed the film at the deaf club soon afterwards. Rochdale Deaf Club's trip to Cleethorpes in 1955 offers a good example of this inclusive process.[37] The trip was captured on film and this was shown in the club the following week. Not only did this allow those who had not travelled the opportunity to see what had taken place but they were also able to view some of the entertainment provided during the evening, when the day out included a visit to Grimsby Deaf Club. An additional benefit for those watching the film was that the conversations and entertainment could be easily accessed, as these took place in sign language. This type of recording and reporting of the club's activities seems to have been a particular feature of Rochdale Deaf Club during this period, as a trip to Great Yarmouth in 1960 was similarly filmed and the results shown soon after the return home.[38] Anecdotal evidence from conversations with deaf club members over a number of years indicates that filming trips, along with a range of other social activities, and showing the results later was not restricted to Rochdale Deaf Club but happened at many deaf clubs in the region and beyond.

Cultural events and outings

Cinema had been a feature of deaf club life from the early part of the twentieth century, with silent films being as popular with deaf viewers as they were for hearing audiences. The use of captions to convey important dialogue or plot developments made silent films equally accessible to deaf viewers. With the advent of the 'talkies', films which still relied heavily on visual humour, such as the comedies of Laurel and Hardy, continued to be shown in deaf clubs throughout the century.[39] Liverpool Deaf Club's inventiveness in showing a series of continental films in 1960 demonstrated the popularity of cinema amongst deaf people and the adaptability of deaf viewers.[40] These films featured English subtitles, which meant they could be enjoyed by a deaf audience, at a time when British and American films were still inaccessible to most deaf people. English language films with subtitles in English were not generally available until many years later, and the first reference in *BDN* to a subtitled English film being shown in a north-west cinema only came in 1980. Bolton Deaf Club seems to have played a major part in broadening access to mainstream entertainment for deaf people in the north west, as some of the first subtitled English language films for deaf audiences were shown in mainstream venues in the town. For example, 'Airport 77' was shown with open subtitles at the town's Octagon Theatre in 1980, and it is interesting to speculate on why the Octagon decided to show a subtitled film for a deaf audience. [41] Either they were responding to an approach from the local deaf club and decided to show the film as a philanthropic exercise or they felt there was a sufficient potential audience to make such a venture financially viable. Whatever the reasons, the Octagon demonstrated their willingness to respond to a deaf audience by becoming one of the pioneers in providing sign language interpreted performances of their programme of plays and shows. This early initiative led to the Octagon eventually providing interpreted performances of all their theatre productions, and their success encouraged other north-west venues to provide similar access for deaf patrons, such as the Duke's Theatre in Lancaster, Preston's Guild Hall and the Oldham Coliseum Theatre.

Perhaps the most notable examples of deaf club members choosing to indulge in what might be considered 'hearing culture' come from Liverpool in the period of the 'Merseybeat' boom of the mid 1960s. *BDN* reported in 1965 that the beat group 'Rory Storm and the Hurricanes' had performed at Liverpool Deaf Club. The evening was deemed to have been such a success that it was hoped to stage a series of these concerts, and later in the year, the group 'The Deejays' performed at the deaf club's Centenary Dinner. [42] Live bands also regularly performed at dinner dances and so certain conceptions of what should or should not be considered as 'deaf culture' are challenged by these examples. Some writers argue that speech has no place in deaf culture; but why then did deaf club members choose to take part in activities that were based almost exclusively on spoken (or in this case, sung) English? [43] In order to have at least partial access – and by extension entertainment – some degree of hearing would seem essential. The answer may be that at least some of those attending the Liverpool concerts were not profoundly deaf; the response must then be that as the event was organised by and for deaf club members, many of those attending must have had some degree of membership of the deaf community. Reports of the Liverpool concerts at least mention that 'suitable amplification' was provided, suggesting that some – if not all – of those present needed enhanced audible access to the concert. Alternatively, it might simply have been that the person reporting the event was unaware that pop groups generally use amplifiers for their performances, and the fact that the venue was a deaf club was immaterial in this respect. Possibly the visual element of the performance, combined with some auditory access, was sufficient to make the event successful for those deaf people present and therefore worth repeating. Another explanation may be that deaf club members were aware of the new fashion in pop music sweeping the city and merely wanted to see what all the fuss was about. Arthur Marwick has acknowledged the emergence of pop and rock music as 'the central cultural phenomenon of the time'.[44] Perhaps it should therefore not be too surprising to learn that deaf people, who are as affected by events in the wider world as anyone else, should be attracted in some way to this cultural revolution taking place within their own city. Whatever the motivations of deaf people in arranging such events, their success – as shown by their repetition – marks them as being integrated into the cultural life of the deaf club and therefore the deaf culture of that particular place and time.

Other leisure activities in the deaf clubs

Trips and visits were by no means the only activity deaf clubs were organising for their members; there were a range of other activities taking place on a regular basis, both in the deaf clubs and elsewhere. Whilst these activities also had cultural connotations simply because of the fact that deaf club members were involved, they were not significantly different from those to be found in many other types of social clubs and voluntary associations.

Dances were normally described in *BDN* as 'dinner dances' and were the second most popular activity in the deaf clubs. As well as dances that were open to all members, there were also a number of celebrations organised by members for family and friends that were marked by a dance. Even comparatively small clubs would organise a variety of events over the Christmas period, with dances held for specific groups such as pensioners, children and youth groups, and deaf/blind members, as well as the more general events. Further evidence of dances at deaf clubs can be found throughout the period and these were often important milestones in clubs' social calendars. From the annual dinner dance held in St Helens in 1945, through the Reunion Dinner Dance held in Lancaster in 1950 which attracted guests from across the north west, to the Manchester Deaf Schools' Reunion Dinner Dance held in 1985, such occasions remained staple items in communal deaf leisure. [45] The numbers involved could often be very high, with 190 present at Blackpool Deaf Club's annual dinner dance in 1965, 210 people attending Lancaster's event in 1975, and 300 at Liverpool Deaf Club's own annual dance.[46]

Dinner dances often added a social dimension to sporting events. A deaf club's annual presentation of sporting trophies usually took place at a dance organised for the occasion, whilst dances were also arranged when another deaf club visited for a sporting contest. When various football teams travelled to Manchester to play matches during 1955, the day was invariably rounded off with a dinner dance in the evening.[47] These were by no means isolated occasions, especially when the opponents or visitors had travelled a long way. Indeed, this was in some ways merely a variation on the visits deaf clubs made to each other as part of a day trip. As these gatherings are almost universally reported as 'dinner dances', with the later addition of references to 'discos', it has to be assumed that music was provided. There are certainly regular references to dancing taking place, and as with the later discos, it seems inconceivable that a dance would be held without music. Just as with the pop group evenings described earlier, deaf people organising social activities that involved sound challenges some of the apparently narrow definitions of deaf cultural activity. In all the above examples of sound playing a part in deaf social life, it must also be remembered that the majority of deaf people are born into hearing families, and so it is not hard to accept that at least some hearing people would also be deaf club members, or at least allowed to join in club activities.

A less contentious means of deaf cultural expression comprised signed plays and dramatic performances. From opposite ends of the period of this study, St Helens Deaf Club's Dinner Dance in 1945 included a series of sketches in sign language and the Deaf Comedians appeared at Preston Deaf Club in 1995, whilst other examples follow later in this chapter.[48] Deaf club members also demonstrated that they were no different than hearing people in the breadth of their interests. All the events one might expect to find in any thriving social club across the north west during the post-war years were also being organised by deaf clubs. Easter bonnet parades, bonfire parties and beauty contests were all regular events and were supplemented by occasional items such as magic shows, April Fools parties and fancy dress parades.[49]

Fundraising has always been a necessary and regular part of deaf club life, as the clubs sought ways to meet the running costs of their premises and activities. Funds were generally needed for redecoration or improvements to the fabric of the deaf clubs, such as installing new kitchens or bars, or to provide holidays for pensioners, children and unemployed members. Even so, it is somewhat surprising to discover that events intended to raise money for the deaf club compromised the third most common type of leisure activity, with fundraising accounting for 15 per cent of deaf club social activity between 1945 and 1995. The immediate post-war period perhaps understandably saw fundraising being a major part of deaf club life, as clubs sought to address the limitations and privations placed on them during the war years. However, rather than reducing as post-war austerity gave way to an economic recovery, fundraising events in deaf clubs increased from the 1960s. Fundraising usually came from one of three main sources: street and pub collections within the local community; a range of sponsored novelty events such as fashion shows, piano pulls and endurance tests organised in the deaf club or by deaf club members; and charitable events organised by local groups on behalf of deaf people in their area. There were numerous examples of these types of fundraising activities

in *British Deaf News* during the post-war period. These included Bolton Deaf
Club holding a Ladies Weekend in 1955 to raise money for new kitchen equipment and Ashton under Lyne Deaf Club organising two Flag Days in 1960
to boost club funds.[50] Bury Deaf Club became one of seventeen charities in
the town to set up a 'good as new' shop in the town centre in 1970, with the
proceeds shared amongst the various groups.[51]

From the mid 1960s onwards, sponsored events became a regular way of
raising money for a whole range of causes and deaf clubs were quick to join
in. The earliest example found was a sponsored walk by Blackburn Deaf Club
in 1970, and reports increased dramatically during the following years. Such
events were also used to raise deaf awareness amongst the local community,
such as Stockport Deaf Club's sponsored Sign Marathon in the local shopping centre in 1985.[52] Contributions to deaf clubs by local charitable bodies
such as Round Tables and Lions Clubs featured regularly in *BDN,* and the
pubs and clubs in Cumbria were especially noticeable as contributors to their
local deaf clubs.[53] In the later years of this study, there was also an increase in
reports of deaf clubs raising money for external appeals and charities. By 1980,
Blackburn Deaf Club's sponsored walk had become an annual event and in an
interesting role reversal, a donation was made to the local Round Table from
the proceeds. The same year saw clubs in the Pendle district donating fifty
pounds to the Blue Peter Appeal for Cambodia.[54] The increase in donations
from deaf clubs may be indicative of a change in attitude amongst members,
from needing or requiring charity towards becoming a provider of support
to other more needy groups. Even so, internal fundraising was still a major
activity, as demonstrated in 1990. The British Deaf Association celebrated
its Centenary that year, and all BDA branches were required to raise money
for the BDA Centenary Appeal, which saw a dramatic increase in fundraising
events reported that year.

There have been strong historical links between the various religious
denominations and deaf clubs, and these links were still in evidence in the late
twentieth century. There were however clear geographical variations in the
reports of church-based activity. Bolton, Southport and Wigan all had a large
proportion of their social and leisure activity linked to religious events, whilst
Preston, Stockport and Warrington report little if any of this type of activity
throughout the fifty years covered by this research. The reasons for this variation are not obvious but there may be a link to the origins of various deaf clubs.
For instance, Preston Deaf Club had strong links with the town's Mary Cross
School, rather than any church, which might help explain the more secular
nature of their activities. On the other hand, there are clear links between religious groups and those deaf clubs that engaged in activities linked to religious

observance. However, it has to be acknowledged that such conclusions are somewhat speculative.

This geographical segregation in religious activity is perhaps best illustrated by the rise in the numbers of deaf choirs during the 1980s and 1990s. These were initially formed to perform hymns and other religious songs in sign language, and these were found exclusively in deaf clubs in the south of the region. Manchester, Liverpool, Wigan and St Helens all boasted deaf choirs from 1980 onwards, and several of these took part in the national Deaf Choirs Festival in Canterbury in 1980.[55] Whatever the reason for the geographical disparity in their popularity, deaf choirs were a regular feature at church services across the north west during the 1980s and 1990s, and demonstrated that religion and church based activities continued to have an influence in the lives of deaf people.

Other deaf club group activities

Deaf clubs provided a range of activities for their members which might be found in other social clubs and voluntary associations and there is nothing intrinsically or uniquely 'deaf' about the types of activities found. Events organised for the eldest and youngest members of the deaf club were a regular part of the programme of activities, which included parties, outings and special events. However, the attraction of deaf clubs for younger and older deaf people underwent significant changes between 1945 and 1995. The number of events arranged for pensioners and older members showed a steady increase, indicating a changing demographic profile of deaf club membership, as a concomitant decline in the number of events for young people showed they were no longer joining deaf clubs. As younger deaf people have become more confident in integrating with the hearing world, so they have been afforded a wider number of opportunities for filling their leisure time. Younger deaf people became less reliant on the deaf club as the hub and provider of their social life, whilst older deaf people remained committed to the more traditional home offered by the deaf club. In many ways the decline in deaf club membership, and the increasingly older age group of those who still attended the clubs, might be seen to reflect a similar decline in other social clubs in the north west. Working-class bases such as political clubs, working men's clubs and trades associations all declined in popularity towards the end of the twentieth century, and deaf clubs were not immune to these wider changes in leisure choices. As disposable income and available leisure time gradually increased for the general population in the post-war years, this corresponded with an increase in the range of activities people could participate in, making the traditional drinking and meeting places less attractive, especially for younger people. However, the impact on the deaf community has been much greater, given the centrality of the deaf club in community life in earlier times.

Conversely, this period of gradually declining membership took place as many of the deaf clubs broadened their range of activities. Many deaf clubs increasingly became centres of learning for their members, particularly in areas of self-help and improvement. One way of informing and educating members was through practical demonstrations and talks, which seem to have been especially popular in the Cumbrian deaf clubs. 1970 was a particularly busy year, with Barrow Deaf Club showing films about Laurel and Hardy (Stan Laurel was born in nearby Ulverston) and the activities of young deaf people. The club also invited a local bank manager to give an interpreted talk to members explaining the new decimal currency which was soon to be introduced, whilst Carlisle Deaf Club were visited by all the local candidates in the forthcoming election to explain their manifestos.[56] Informative and educational talks given to deaf club members in Cumbria during 1975 included a first aid demonstration by the St John's Ambulance service; a cookery demonstration by the local electricity board; insights into forensic investigations from an Inspector from the Cumbrian Constabulary; the work of the Royal National Lifeboat Institute and the role of the deaf psychiatric unit at Whittingham Hospital near Preston.[57] More talks and demonstrations seem to have taken place in Cumbria than in any other part of the north west, although many similar examples were found from other deaf clubs.

The other main avenue for providing an increased range of social, self-help and educational activities was through societies and courses. As well as national bodies such as the Deaf Camping and Caravanning Club and the Deaf Motorists Club, fell walking groups were established in both Kendal (on the edge of the Lake district) and Manchester (close to both the Lake and Peak Districts), and attracted members from across the country. [58] A whole range of local self-help and interest groups were set up, with keep fit classes, film and photography clubs and drama groups being particularly popular. Drama groups were a feature of many deaf clubs, with a wide range of plays being produced, and these were usually presented in sign language, as the most appropriate means of communication for both the actors and those watching the plays. The choice of certain plays raises some interesting questions about how these plays were translated from English into sign language, and by whom. For example, Liverpool Deaf Club's Drama Group seems to have been particularly active and thriving in the 1960s and 1970s. *A Midsummer Night's Dream* was presented in 1970, following their earlier production of *Oedipus Rex* in 1960. [59] In both instances the plays were signed, with the 1960 play having a spoken narration provided 'for hearing friends'.[60] The language of these plays is not necessarily easily accessible or understood by hearing audiences, and the translation of the plays into sign language must have been a long and difficult process. The adaptation of the 1960 play was undertaken by the Assistant Supervisor of the local Deaf Society, a hearing person presumably sufficiently proficient in sign language to translate the text in a meaningful way.

Liverpool was by no means the only deaf club taking part in drama productions, but they do appear to have been the most adventurous in their choice of productions. No doubt the same group's productions of the pantomimes *Mother Goose* and *Peter Pan* (both of which included singing and dancing) in 1970 proved less arduous in terms of translation.[61]

Away from the stage, deportment, make-up and hairstyling classes were provided in Bolton in 1960.[62] Several keep fit and aerobics classes were set up in various clubs, and many clubs had groups for unemployed members, mothers and toddlers and ladies Groups.[63] In the 1990s, 'Triangle Clubs' for lesbian and gay deaf people reflected the increasing acceptance of minority groups in wider society, as did the establishment of a deaf Asians group in Manchester in 1995.[64] Educational ventures for deaf people included further education classes provided by Rochdale Deaf Club in 1965, reading and writing classes in Warrington in 1975, and Liverpool Deaf Club organised a training course for unemployed deaf people to become sign language tutors in 1995.[65]

Deaf club members also began to take a more active role in events amongst the wider community during the post-war years. When this involvement included some degree of success for a deaf person or reflected well on the deaf community, then the news was passed on to other deaf people through the pages of *British Deaf News*. Thus the achievement of a deaf man in winning the 'Best Decorated Car in Morecambe Carnival' competition three years running was reported in *BDN* with a degree of pride, as was the presence of a couple from Blackburn Deaf Club at a Buckingham Palace garden party in 1990.[66] The couple, accompanied by sign language interpreters, were being rewarded for their work with the deaf club and as members of the local deaf church. The growth in reports may also be indicative of the growing integration of deaf people into wider society, resulting from a growing confidence amongst deaf people in meeting hearing people. Sign language users were no longer isolated in the deaf clubs, as deaf awareness grew and deaf people became less hidden away due to changes in education policy. Following the Warnock Report of 1978, segregated education for deaf pupils was largely replaced by integration into mainstream schools, and whilst sign language as an educational medium remained very much in the minority, the use of sign language in public places increased as deaf people attained a higher profile than they had when they were hidden away in deaf schools.

Sport in the deaf clubs

In addition to serving as providers of various leisure activities for local deaf people, the deaf clubs acted as the venues and bases for a number of team and individual sports. This provision was well established in north-west England by 1945, as the region had played a leading role in organising sport for deaf people and formalising its administration.

Organised deaf sport in north-west England developed from the Lancashire Deaf and Dumb Orme League, which was founded in 1924 by a group of deaf billiards players. Named after a local billiards manufacturing company, who provided the shield presented to the winners, the league developed from a number of deaf individuals initially arranging a series of friendly matches. Eventually shortening its name to the more manageable Orme League, the success of the competition led to demands for other sports to be included, and in 1947, the North West Deaf Sports Association (NWDSA) was formed to oversee a wider range of sporting activity. Acting as the regional body of the British Deaf Amateur Sports Association, the NWDSA organised a number of sporting events across the north west throughout the post-war period. The NWDSA was also instrumental in setting up the highly successful Indoor Sports League which was the mainstay of many deaf clubs' sporting activities through the winter months. From the original focus on billiards, the NWDSA eventually came to encompass darts, whist, pool, football, snooker, dominoes, badminton, squash, cricket and swimming competitions.[67] The NWDSA became the North West Deaf Sports Council in the early 1980s, as part of the changes that saw the national body become the British Deaf Sports Council. These organisations were concerned solely with the organisation and control of competition between deaf competitors. Neither organisation had any control over deaf sportsmen and women competing against hearing opponents. Deaf sport thus has important political implications, as Padden and Humphreys acknowledge: 'sports organisations like these are one of the few places where deaf people exercise almost total control over their own affairs, from deciding their own rules to determining who qualifies as a member'.[68]

BDN reported deaf sporting events and achievements throughout the twentieth century, with news appearing in the dedicated sports pages and amongst the reports from deaf clubs. A total of 573 separate reports were found in the period 1945 to 1995, although this does not fully reflect the overall level of sporting activity. This is due to the distinctive nature of sports reporting when compared to leisure activity; a report on leisure related to a specific event, whereas a report on sport often referred to the participation of a team or individual in a league or cup competition. This naturally meant that participants were involved in many individual matches or contests, which greatly exceeded the number of actual reports.

The range of deaf club-based sport

The range of sports reported by north-west deaf club members was comparatively narrow, with only eleven sports featuring with any regularity. These were:

Table 5 The range of deaf club-based sports

Outdoor sports	Indoor sports
Football (18%)	Dominoes (8%)
Cricket (5%)	Snooker/billiards/pool (26%)
Athletics (1%)	Darts (14%)
Bowls (18%)	Chess (4%)
	Badminton (1%)
	Table Tennis (3%)
	Swimming (2%)

There were isolated instances of other sports taking place but the overwhelming majority of reports were restricted to the eleven mainstream sports outlined above. Of these, three sports (snooker, football and bowls) accounted for 62 per cent of reported sporting activity during the research period; when the figures for darts are added, these four sports made up 76 per cent of the sporting activity of deaf club members.

The majority of deaf sporting activity took place indoors, with outdoor sport mainly restricted to football in winter and bowls in summer, with some limited evidence of cricket and athletics. There were numerous examples of indoor sporting leagues being organised during the research period and indoor sports events provided the basis for informal but regular social gatherings. These events took place both in the deaf clubs and in other venues, with opponents including both deaf and hearing competitors. When these sporting events involved deaf opponents, they appear to have been treated as much as social events as sporting contests. On the other hand, there is little evidence to suggest that organised socialising formed a major or regular part of sporting competitions between deaf and hearing opponents. The participation of deaf teams and players in local leagues was the norm rather than their playing solely with and against other deaf teams. Some sports appear more 'inter-deaf' than others; for example, reports concerning chess, table tennis and athletics seem to be restricted almost exclusively to matches and contests against other deaf people. There is very little evidence of deaf clubs taking part in these particular activities against hearing opponents, rare examples being Blackburn and Oldham Deaf Clubs' membership of local table tennis leagues in 1960 and 1995 respectively.[69] Rochdale Deaf Club's table tennis team winning the championship of their local league in 1960 was an even more rare example of a deaf team achieving success in a mixed setting.[70] Although deaf individuals also joined hearing teams and clubs, there is little evidence of such involvement unless the individual concerned achieved some success.

Trends in sports participation

Before looking at deaf people's involvement in individual sports, some general trends in popularity and participation can be identified. Determining the comparative popularity of various sports is to some extent problematic, especially when based on data that may appear solely quantitative. Nevertheless, it is possible to reach some general conclusions based on the number of reports in *BDN*, which also provide some qualitative insights into the value placed on different sports. It seems logical to assume that deaf club members would not take part in sports they did not like and therefore reports of these sports would not appear in *BDN*. However, there are some instances that show that deaf people were participating in certain sports, but this participation was not reported.

The most reported activity was playing snooker and billiards, with 168 reports between 1945 and 1995. The Orme League was based in deaf clubs, indicating that many (if not all) clubs possessed at least one snooker table, despite needing adequate space and the expense of buying a table. It is also interesting to speculate on the acceptance of snooker by the Missioners, given the attitude towards snooker and snooker halls by many religious groups. The notion of prowess at the game indicating a 'misspent youth' does not seem to have been applied to deaf club members. Indeed, it could be suggested that the Missioners may have been actively promoting the playing snooker and billiards in the deaf clubs, as a means of keeping young deaf people out of the snooker halls. Pool began to feature during the 1970s, as the game gained a foothold in the nation's leisure time generally. Football was only the third most popular activity with 120 reports, just behind bowls with 121 reports.

The less energetic nature of the two most popular sports may indicate a comparatively high average age of deaf club members. Changes in the welfare provision for deaf people also impacted on the recruitment of new members into the deaf clubs. The consequences for deaf sports teams were that as players became older, there was not necessarily a succession of younger players to replace them. The comparative popularity of snooker, bowls and darts in the latter years of this research supports the notion that the average age of deaf club members was increasing.

Of the eleven sports found in *BDN* reports from north-west England, some hardly ever appeared, with badminton and athletics only featuring fourteen times between them. There is no evidence of deaf people taking part in organised athletics events below county or regional levels, whilst golf and squash, which experienced a huge growth in Britain during the 1970s and 1980s, were rarely reported in the north west, although there is evidence that deaf people were taking up these sports. This was certainly the case with golf, which despite the lack of reports in *BDN*, had a strong following in the north west in the latter years covered by this research. The English Deaf Golf Association (EDGA), founded in the early 1980s, held its annual National Championship in north-west England, and the majority of the English deaf golf team came from the region. The national team competed in international competitions, including the World Deaf Golf Championships.[71] Based solely on the evidence provided by *BDN*, it is not possible to state with any degree of certainty which other sports individual deaf people were taking part in nor to what extent. What can be said is that those taking part were not representing their local deaf clubs in competition with hearing opponents, nor were their activities being reported as such in *British Deaf News*. Therefore, this participation cannot be considered as part of the communal sporting life of the deaf clubs, although it was no doubt of interest and importance to those involved and offered some personal satisfaction.

The individual sports enjoyed by deaf club members

Having identified some trends in sporting involvement by deaf people, it is worth spending some time on a brief analysis of the individual sports found in *British Deaf News*. Snooker and billiards and in later years, pool collectively constituted the most popular activity, representing 26 per cent of all reported sport amongst deaf club members. Many deaf billiards players played in the Orme League, and snooker was also very popular in deaf clubs; both games were mainstays of the Indoor Games League.[72] Many deaf clubs were also active in their local leagues, playing against hearing teams, with several examples of deaf club teams gaining success. A member of Oldham Deaf Club reached the final of the local billiards competition in 1965, whilst nearby Manchester Deaf Club won both the snooker and the billiards leagues they entered in 1970, in which they competed against hearing teams.[73] Deaf players sometimes tested their skills against touring professionals, as when John Parrott took part in a charity event in Lancaster Deaf Club in 1985.[74] Parrott's fellow professional Willie Thorne gave a demonstration of trick shots and played against members of Kendal Deaf Club's snooker team in 1995.[75]

The apparently sedate sport of snooker could also be the cause of some tension between deaf and hearing people. A report in *British Deaf News* in 1975 included a complaint from Warrington Deaf Club that the snooker team had been fined fifty pence by the local hearing league they played in for the late arrival of results. The deaf club's claim that the results had been posted in time failed to impress the league's committee, who refused to accept the claim that the letter had taken four days to travel two miles. A much more serious complaint followed, when the club reported they were being repeatedly fined for non-attendance at meetings of the league. The club felt they were being unfairly treated, as they were unable to arrange or afford for an interpreter to attend the meetings. Apologies for their absence were sent, together with an explanation of the situation, but still the fines were levied.[76] This instance shows that many of the frustrations faced by deaf people in daily life, often due to a lack of awareness or understanding on the part of hearing people, could also affect them in their leisure time.

Bowls was the major summer sport for deaf club members, and again many clubs were active and successful both in local hearing leagues and in exclusively deaf competitions. Bowls also occasionally afforded deaf people the opportunity to succeed in the sporting world in non-competitive ways, and these successes were celebrated with as much pride as any sporting achievement. When a Manchester deaf man was elected President of the Lancashire Bowling League in 1960, this was a source of pride for all connected with his deaf club. The news was reported as a major achievement not only for the deaf individual concerned, but also for the wider deaf community. Manchester Deaf Club's claim to be the only deaf team in the English Bowling Association was a similar cause for pride and celebration.[77] Such successes served as an antidote to the less positive aspects of involvement with hearing sport illustrated by the experience of the Warrington deaf snooker team.

Football was the most popular outdoor sport for deaf club members in winter; indeed, it was the only outdoor winter sport that the majority of deaf clubs took part in. There is ample evidence of deaf teams playing against both deaf and hearing opponents, whether in local leagues or in competitions exclusively for deaf teams. The Lancashire Deaf Football League was in existence in 1945, and Burnley, Preston, Rochdale and Bolton were all members of the league in that year.[78] In subsequent years, the North West Deaf Sports Council ran a football competition for the clubs in the area, and teams also entered the national cup competition organised by the British Deaf Sports Council. Virtually all the deaf teams also took part in their local hearing leagues, as well as five-a-side competitions. Deaf leagues only featured a few teams, meaning fewer fixtures, and the standard could be quite variable.[79] By playing in a local league, deaf teams could guarantee a greater number of matches, and find an appropriate level at which to play. Hearing football was also perceived to be of a higher standard, and so could take precedence over involvement in deaf sport, as shown by the actions of Blackburn Deaf Club in 1960. Rather than join the winter deaf sports league, Blackburn's younger members chose instead to enter a team in one of the town's football leagues.[80] The sporting attractions of regular football against hearing opponents was obviously greater than the social and sporting attractions of darts, snooker and card games against deaf opponents.

Darts and dominoes were the subject of regular reports in *BDN*, and both were standard components, alongside snooker and billiards, of the various deaf indoor sports leagues in the north west. There were matches and competitions for both men and women and once again deaf players and teams joined local leagues to play with and against hearing opponents. These events were hosted in local pubs and clubs, as well as in deaf clubs, indicating the way in which various sports could serve as a means of integrating deaf and hearing competitors in shared competition.

Cricket was the only outdoor summer sport other than bowls that deaf sportsmen were regularly involved in. In terms of the number of reports found, cricket was less popular than dominoes, and there is very little evidence of much involvement at club level, although there were annual inter-regional matches featuring north-west players. For example, there were regular Lancashire versus Yorkshire 'Roses' matches throughout the 1950s and 1960s, with Lancashire County Cricket Club's Old Trafford ground being the venue on more than one occasion. The report of the 1960 match begins, 'Once again, the Lancashire County Cricket Club has very kindly permitted the use of the County Ground …' suggesting the ground had previously been used for this fixture.[81] There is some evidence of a north-west deaf cricket league in existence in 1985, which may have involved as many as seven deaf clubs or as few as four; clubs played six matches each but it is not clear whether return home and away fixtures were played, or if opponents played each other just once.[82] The lack of evidence from either 1980 or 1990 suggests that the league was a short-lived enterprise that could not be sustained.

Cricket formed part of the sporting life of the deaf schools in the area and beyond, but how much this involvement was due to compulsion rather than choice might be open to debate. Certainly participation in cricket did not continue to any great extent when deaf people graduated into the deaf clubs. Perhaps one disincentive for deaf participation at club level was the cost of equipment, and as with other sports, the level of technical skill and coaching required to play at a decent standard may have also dissuaded deaf people from taking up the game. As with all deaf sport, the lack of numbers to form teams was undoubtedly a major factor; as was the cost of having to travel to find opponents if there were none available locally. There were also no reports found of deaf cricketers playing for hearing teams, although this cannot be taken as definite proof that deaf individuals did not join hearing cricket clubs.

Other deaf club sporting and competitive activity

Chess was very popular from well before the Second World War, with gambits and discussions of matches featuring in each issue of *British Deaf Times* in the pre-war years. This interest continued after the war, and the north west was particularly blessed with chess players; the entire England team for the match against Scotland in 1950 was drawn from the north west.[83] There was an active north-west league in 1950 featuring teams from eight deaf clubs.[84] However, in terms of reports in *BDN*, the game suffered a rapid post-war decline after having been the second most popular activity in 1955. Nevertheless, the game did not die out completely, with *British Deaf News* running a national correspondence league for many years after 1950, which included members from north-west deaf clubs.[85] Two Liverpool Deaf Club members travelled to play in the World Deaf Chess Championships in Germany in 1955, whilst the English Deaf Championships attracted forty players to Preston in 1975.[86] As with so many other deaf sporting events, even a chess tournament could be the basis for organising a social gathering, with 240 people attended the celebratory dinner that followed the 1975 championship. The number of people involved in these later events also suggests that whilst the number of reports may have decreased, there were still significant numbers engaging in chess matches between deaf people.[87]

Athletics featured during the summer months at regional and national levels, but there is no evidence of inter-club meetings. Given the small number of potential competitors in each club, the costs of specialist equipment and the need for a suitable venue, the staging of formal athletics events was almost certainly not feasible at club level. There is some evidence of local events taking place in other parts of Britain, such as the annual walking race in Hull reported in 1955, but these were not large scale athletics meetings.[88] There were regular meetings at county and regional level, however; examples of meetings at various levels were found in most years from 1955 to 1985.[89] Athletes from north-west deaf clubs were amongst those who attended the trials to select the team for the 1965 World Games for the Deaf.[90]

Badminton was certainly a feature of the sporting life of deaf people in other parts of the country, as shown by the existence of both cup and league competitions in London in 1945.[91] However, badminton does not appear to have been especially strong in the north west, with only ten reports from the entire research period. However, the lack of reports may well hide the true extent of participation, as reports in 1985 refer to a north-west badminton knock-out competition.[92] This suggests that there were enough individual deaf people involved in the sport at that time to make a local knock-out competition a viable proposition, although this does not appear to have survived for very long or involved many players.

Swimming was another sport that was only occasionally mentioned in the reports from north-west deaf clubs. The majority of these appeared during the 1980s, with little other evidence from before or after this period. Both Manchester and Southport Deaf Clubs boasted medal winners at the National Championships of 1980, whilst the National Championships were held in Wigan in 1985.[93] *BDN* reported in the same year that the North West Championships were being held for the first time since 1957, and it was also noted that all the officials at the event would be deaf for the first time.[94] Once again, sport provided deaf people with an opportunity to travel, when members from several north-west deaf clubs were included in the Great Britain team which travelled to the European Deaf Swimming Championships in Antibes.[95] Water sport was also the source of local and national deaf pride when the selection of an eighteen-year-old member of Lancaster Deaf Club for the England Youth Water Polo team was reported in 1980. The pride was due to his being the only deaf member of the team, but the reporter also chose to conclude the report with the following comment: 'well done, Steven, that's another achievement against the hearing world ....'.[96] This seems a somewhat inappropriate comment in a report which otherwise expressed pride at the young man's achievement in being selected on his ability, rather than being excluded because of his deafness. Perhaps this illustrates the underlying tension felt by many deaf people when they find themselves in direct competition with hearing people, even when that competition was for places on the same team.

Missing sports

There are some notable omissions from the record of deaf people's involvement in various sports. Nationally popular sports such as netball, squash and angling taking place in the north west hardly ever featured in *BDN*, with only three reports of deaf angling contests, two reports relating to netball and nothing at all concerning squash.[97] This is despite both sports being included in the activities of the North West Deaf Sports Council.[98] Indeed, a report from Bolton in 1995 specifically refers to the club winning the NWDSC netball championship.[99] Although reports on these sports may have appeared in other years not covered by this research, the general lack of coverage suggests that these were not major participant sports for deaf people. Another factor is the need for specialist equipment and venues for sports such as netball, squash and tennis. Deaf people in the north west may well have been joining hearing clubs as individuals, rather than joining as a group or team of deaf people. The possible reasons for this can be addressed by looking again at deaf people's involvement in golf, for which more evidence is available. As was mentioned above, golf did not feature at all in the reports of north-west deaf sport from 1945 to 1995. However, deaf people were most certainly joining local golf clubs. Evidence provided by the British Deaf Golf Association indicates that deaf golfers of higher ability joined clubs on an individual basis, and played largely with and against hearing golfers.[100] These players improved their handicaps as a result of playing at a higher level, although the social rewards were somewhat reduced for those who had difficulty communicating with their playing partners. The greater the degree of integration, the less likely that such golfers would have their activities reported in *BDN*, as this activity was not part of the communal life of the deaf club. Those who preferred to join golf clubs in the company of other deaf players tended to socialise less outside of their immediate group (i.e. with hearing golfers), but gained greater social benefits from playing in the company of their deaf contemporaries. A consequence of this restricted competition was that deaf social golfers did not develop their skills to the same extent and so typically had a higher handicap than their more integrated fellow deaf golfers. Both instances involved making a decision on what was the greater motivation for playing the game – the social rewards or the sporting rewards. For those deaf golfers who had limited communication with hearing people, it appears (as with other sports) that it was not possible to reap both types of benefit fully. The lack of social rewards may have deterred many potential deaf golfers from taking up the game, when they could not do so in the company of those who could provide the social life, which is an important part of sports participation.

There were a number of sports that were particularly associated with the north west in the post-war period, such as greyhound racing, pigeon racing and Rugby League. However, there is no evidence in the years surveyed to indicate any organised deaf club involvement in these activities, either as participants or observers. Rugby League as a participant sport would no doubt be subject to the same pressures as football in terms of available players, finance, facilities and equipment. Research has shown that as the officiating of football matches relies heavily on sound, this can cause problems for deaf players.[101] In both codes of rugby, the referee communicates his instructions to players mainly by word of mouth, which is vital to the smooth flowing of the game; visual signals are only given once a decision has been made. Therefore, finding alternative ways of controlling the game to accommodate deaf players may have been a disincentive to encouraging deaf players to become involved. Even after the introduction of a formalised system of signalling decisions in recent years, rugby has remained a rarity in deaf sport. Without suitably qualified coaches able to communicate the often complex technical details and rules of the game to players who could not hear, the lack of participation in the game by deaf people is perhaps not surprising.

The lack of any organised deaf group involvement in greyhound racing or pigeon racing seems to fit into a broader trend of non-participation in certain sporting events. There is no evidence to indicate that deaf club members made organised group trips to mainstream sporting events as spectators. For example, there were a number of greyhound tracks in the region during the post-war years, but there were no reports of any visits being made to greyhound meetings. Racecourses in the north-west include Cartmel and Carlisle in Cumbria, Haydock Park near Wigan and Aintree in Liverpool. There are also several more within easy travelling distance, such as those in Chester and Uttoxeter. Only one report of a visit to a race meeting was found, when Blackpool Deaf Club members made a trip to Chester Races in 1990.[102] Not even the Grand National meetings in Liverpool seemed to have been sufficiently attractive to warrant a deaf club outing during the years of this research. One factor that may have mitigated against deaf people attending any type of race meeting was the importance of gambling in these events. As Richard Holt has shown, betting on the results of races (whether legally or illegally) was a central part of the attraction of these sporting activities.[103] The influence of religious groups in all aspects of deaf life, particularly that of the Missioner based in the deaf clubs and societies, may well have been a major reason why these sports are missing from the record of deaf club organised activities. This is not to say that deaf people did not attend race meetings of all types on an individual basis, or indeed wager on the outcome of races, but if they did, they were careful not to advertise the fact through the pages of *British Deaf News*.

Perhaps surprisingly, there were no reports of trips to professional football matches, despite the popularity amongst deaf club members of football as a participant sport. There was a high number of football clubs in the area, with as many as twenty north-west clubs playing in the Football League at various times during the research period, as well as a myriad of semi-professional clubs at lower levels. Attendance at cricket matches was another activity for which there is no evidence of organised deaf participation, despite the post-war popularity of county and Test cricket (both of which were held at the Old Trafford ground in Manchester) and the particular attraction of league cricket in north-west towns. Lancashire County Cricket Club also regularly played matches in Liverpool, Blackpool, Lytham and Southport. Therefore deaf people were not short of opportunities to attend cricket matches, but there is no evidence that they were doing so in large numbers. From the lack of evidence, it would appear that attendance at mainstream sporting outings was not something that deaf club members did as an organised club activity.

There are several possible conclusions to be drawn from this lack of reports: firstly, deaf people attended such events as individuals or in small groups, but not as part of an organised deaf club event; or secondly, organised trips did take place but were not thought worthy of reporting. These activities were adequately provided for throughout the north west, and so anyone from the local deaf community with an interest in these pursuits could find ample opportunities to take part. They could easily go along to a football or cricket match, or visit a racecourse or greyhound track, without the need to plan the event in advance. A third alternative of course is that deaf people simply were not interested in these activities and so chose not to attend, which would at least explain the almost total lack of evidence to suggest that they did. The comparative lack of cricket matches involving deaf teams may at least partly explain the apparent lack of trips to Old Trafford. However, the same lack of participation as a reason for not watching professional matches does not apply to football and it is unrealistic to suggest deaf people did not attend football matches. Whatever the true reason for the lack of evidence on these sports, some interesting questions about why deaf people chose certain sports to participate in and not others are worthy of further examination.

The role of leisure and sport in the deaf community

Leisure and sport have played a central role in bringing deaf people together in north-west England, and as a result helped to both construct and maintain the deaf community in the region and act as a medium for its cultural expression. Various events were regularly used as a vehicle (often indeed as an excuse) for wider socialising between deaf clubs. Such events brought deaf people together not just locally, but also on a number of ever-wider geographical levels, up to and including international exchanges. The ways in which deaf people in north-west England engaged in leisure practices and the benefits they gained from doing so did not differ significantly from what was going on in other parts of Britain. Different patterns of leisure preferences might be found in other regions; Scots for example may have been more involved in religious events, whilst deaf clubs in more isolated areas of the country may have taken fewer trips to neighbouring clubs. No matter how the specific details may have varied, it is clear that deaf people across the UK were brought together by their shared deafness and they gained great sociological and psychological rewards from doing so. The sheer number of occasions that deaf people sought each other out, whether as the primary motivation for an event or just as an adjunct to a day out, shows the importance that shared leisure has played in developing and maintaining a sense of community amongst deaf people. Deaf leisure in north-west England was not unique in either the deaf experience or within the context of wider leisure practices within the region. Deaf people in this part of the country were doing exactly the same as their hearing neighbours and for precisely the same reasons. There was nothing especially 'deaf' about the ways they chose to spend their leisure time. That they did some of these things more often than their hearing contemporaries merely shows how much attachment was placed on them. Nor were they doing anything that was significantly differ-ent to other deaf people across the country; there is no evidence to suggest that there was a distinct north-west deaf leisure culture. Indeed, the number of trips into and out of the region and the participation of north-west deaf clubs members in communal holidays with deaf people from other parts of the coun-try indicates that there were many more commonalities than differences.

The breadth and levels of activity outlined in this chapter emphasise the social function of deaf clubs. This role involved not just the local deaf popula-tion but also served as a means of bringing deaf people together with others from outside the immediate locality. Deaf clubs were much more than simply a place where like-minded people met to drink and socialise for a few hours. For many deaf people, deaf clubs formed the hub of their lives and provided a refuge from the pressures of everyday life. In addition, deaf clubs allowed their members to escape from the specific pressures associated with being a member of a largely misunderstood minority who were socially and linguistically isolated from interaction with the surrounding majority culture. The way in which deaf people chose to take part in certain leisure activities may have been no different from any other members of society. However, there were some aspects of deaf leisure activity, particularly those communal events organ-ised and shared by deaf club members, which served a uniquely deaf cultural purpose. Precisely what an understanding of these shared leisure and sporting activities tells us about the nature of the deaf community will be discussed in the concluding chapter.

Notes

1   *BDT*, 1950, pp. 117, 119
2   *BDT*, 1950, p. 18
3   *BDN*, 1960, p. 40; 1970, p. 222
4   *BDN*, 1980, p. 393
5   *BDN*, 1965, p. 76; 1990, September, p. 20; December, p. 24
6   *BDN*, 1955, p. 150
7   *BDN*, 1985, January, p. 17; 1995, May, p. 23
8   *BDN*, 1985, September, p. 23; November, p. 15; 1990, July, p. 19; October, p. 65
9   *BDN*, 1995, August, p. 23
10 Woll, B., 'International perspectives on sign language communication', *International Journal of Sign Linguistics* 1, 2 (1990), pp. 107–120
11 *BDN*, 1955, p. 150
12 *BDN*, 1955, p. 152
13 *BDN*, 1970, p. 305
14 *BDN*, 1975, p. 87; 1985, April, p. 16
15 *BDN*, 1970, p. 307; 1975, p. 158.
16 *BDN*, 1985, November, p. 15
17 *BDN*, 1990, July, p. 19; August, p. 19
18 *BDN*, 1960, p. 67; 1965, p. 75; 1970, pp. 191, 308; 1995, August, p. 21; November, p. 21
19 *BDN*, 1960, p. 93
20 *BDN*, 1965, p. 257
21 *BDN*, 1975, p. 19; 1980, p. 234
22 *BDN*, 1970, p. 305; 1975, p. 159; 1975, p. 157
23 *BDN*, 1975, p. 28
24 *BDN*, 1990, January, p. 21; June, p. 16; September, p. 18; November, p. 19
25 *BDN*, 1990, January, p. 17; June, p. 16
26 *BDN*, 1990, April, p. 22; May, p. 21; August, p. 24; December, p. 27; 1995, May, p. 21; September, p. 23; October, p. 24
27 *BDN*, 1960, p. 59
28 *BDN*, 1970, p. 155
29 *BDN*, 1955, p. 152; 1960, p. 93
30 BDN, 1965, pp. 65, 72, 75; 1990, May, p. 20
31 Barton, S., *Working class organisations and popular tourism, 1840–1970* (Manchester: Manchester University Press, 2005)
32 *BDN*, 1995, July, p. 21; October, p. 23
33 *BDN*, 1990, October p. 21–25 *passim*
34 *BDN*, 1965, pp. 23, 65; 1975, pp. 88, 158, 159
35 For example, see *BDN*, 1980, p. 422
36 *BDN*, 1970, p. 273
37 *BDN*, 1955, p. 122
38 *BDN*, 1960, p. 65

39   For example Salford Deaf Club held fortnightly film shows *BDN*, 1955, January/
      February, p. 28

40   *BDN*, 1960, pp. 89–90

41   *BDN*, 1980, p. 421

42   *BDN* 1965, p. 255

43   For example Padden, 'The deaf community and deaf culture', p. 42

44   Marwick, A., 'The arts, books, media and entertainments in Britain since 1945'
      in J. Obelkevich and P. Catterall (eds), *Understanding post-war British society*
      (London, Routledge, 1994), p. 187

45   *BDT*, 1945, January/February, p. 20; 1950, January/February, p. 19; *BDN*, 1985,
      November, p. 18

46   *BDN*, 1960, p. 14; 1975, pp. 49, 50

47   *BDN*, 1955, p. 28

48   *BDT*, 1945, January/February, p. 20; *BDN*, 1995, December, p. 24

49   See for example *BDN*, 1955, p. 124; 1960, p. 15; 1970, p. 227; 1975, pp. 88–89;
      1980, p. 349; 1985, p. 13; 1995, January, p. 27

50   *BDN*, 1955, p. 88; 1960, p. 13

51   *BDN*, 1970, p. 156

52   *BDN*, 1970, p. 220; 1985, September, p. 21

53   Examples can be found in *BDN*, 1955, pp. 26, 150; 1980, pp. 355, 393

54   *BDN*, 1980, pp. 235, 344

55   *BDN*, 1980, p. 234

56   *BDN*, 1970, pp. 155, 220, 263

57   *BDN*, 1975, pp. 92, 120, 161, 185

58   *BDN*, 1965, p. 256; 1985, May, p. 11, November, p. 15; 1990, January, p. 17; 1995,
      December, p. 24

59   *BDN*, 1960, p. 42; 1970, p. 227

60   *BDN*, 1960, p. 42

61   *BDN*, 1970, p. 160, 227

62   *BDN*, 1960, p. 85

63   *BDN*, 1960, p. 39; 1975, pp. 159, 160, 183; 1985, February, p. 15; March, p. 15;
      July, p. 18

64   *BDN*, 1995, February, p. 25; September, p. 23

65   *BDN*, 1965, p. 297; 1975, p. 192; 1995, April, p. 24

66   *BDN*, 1980, p. 349; 1990, pp. 20, 21

67   *BDN*, 1984 August, p. 24; Scarfe, L. (ed.), *A brief history of the NWDSC*
      (Manchester, North West Deaf Sports Council, 1996)

68   C. Padden and T. Humphries, *Deaf in America: voices from a culture* (London:
      Harvard University Press, 1988), p. 49

69   *BDN* 1960, p. 85; 1990, June, p. 20

70   *BDN* 1960, p. 43

71   Stuart Harrison, Development Office of the British Deaf Golf Association, in
      personal communication with the author

72   *BDT*, 1945, p. 119; *BDN*, 1955, p. 156; 1960, p. 59

73   *BDN*, 1965, p. 296; 1970, p. 268

74   *BDN*, 1985, December, p. 18

75   *BDN*, 1995, July p. 23

76   *BDN*, 1975, p. 128. Deaf football clubs reported similar experiences with ruling bodies not making allowances for the particular needs of deaf footballers. See Atherton *et al.*, *Deaf United*, pp. 88–89

77   *BDN*, 1960, p. 64

78   *BDT*, 1945, p. 38

79   For a fuller history of deaf football, see Atherton *et al.*, *Deaf United* and Paull, A., 'The establishment of the English Deaf Football Council, 1983', *Deaf History Journal* 6, 1 (2001) pp. 14–15

80   *BDN*, 1960, p. 85

81   *BDT*, 1945, p. 96; 1960, p. 63

82   *BDN*, 1985: July, p. 18; September, p. 18

83   *BDT*, 1950, pp. 14, 33

84   *BDT*, 1950 p. 34

85   *BDT*, 1950, p. 14; 1960, p. 36 are just two examples

86   *BDN*, 1955, p. 58; 1975, p. 28

87   Boyce, A. 'History of the I.C.S.C.', *Deaf History Journal* Supplement V (2002) pp. 19–22; Gardner, P., 'British deaf chess history', *Deaf History Journal* Supplement III (2002) pp. 7–10

88   *BDN*, 1955, pp. 106–107

89   *BDN*, 1955, pp. 112–113; *BDN* 1960, p. 56

90   *BDN*, 1965, Spring, p. 256; Autumn, p. 26

91   *BDT*, 1945, pp. 58, 115

92   *BDN*, 1985 March, p. 13

93   *BDN*, 1980, p. 339; 1985, May, pp. 18–19

94   *BDN*, 1985 May, p. 20

95   *BDN*, 1985 March, pp. 19–20

96   *BDN*, 1980, p. 349

97   *BDN*, 1970, pp. 191, 266 (angling); 1985, April, p. 17 (netball); 1995, July, p. 21 (angling); 1995 August, p. 21 (netball)

98   Scarfe, *A brief history of the NWDSC*

99   *BDN*, 1995, August p. 21

100   Harrison, personal communication with author

101   Atherton *et al.*, *Deaf United* includes a discussion of the adaptations made in the officiating of matches involving deaf players

102   *BDN*, 1990 September, p. 18

103   Holt, *Sport and the British*, pp. 179–194

9

LEISURE IN THE DEAF COMMUNITY: MORE THAN JUST PASSING THE TIME

When I set out on this research, I was seeking to answer some basic questions about deaf people, their community and the ways they interacted with each other. I knew this interaction was largely based in the network of deaf clubs to be found around the country but there was little evidence of what these communal activities involved or what importance deaf people placed upon them, other than some vague generalisations. I believe I have now found the answers to the questions I posed myself, in that I have discovered how many deaf clubs there were in the post-war United Kingdom and where they were located. As part of this process, the leisure choices of deaf club members have been uncovered, answering the key question of 'What exactly did deaf people do in these clubs?' As well as answering these essentially quantitative questions, the insights this study has provided into the lived experiences of deaf people in the UK since 1945 has also revealed the importance of these activities in the wider social and cultural life of deaf people in Britain. This in turn has demonstrated the role involvement in leisure activities has played in the formation and maintenance of a distinct deaf community in Britain. Therefore, what has been learnt about how deaf people chose to spend their free time, with whom, where and how often will be briefly revisited here. In addition, the ways in which a closer understanding of deaf people's involvement in communal leisure challenges some of the negative perceptions of deaf people that have been dominant throughout history will also be addressed. What the future might hold for the deaf clubs will comprise the concluding discussion of this book.

Firstly, it is clear that deaf club members had a busy and varied social life, and in this way they were no different to similar social and voluntary groups in the hearing world. If anything, the sheer volume of social activities taking place under the auspices of the deaf clubs suggests their members enjoyed a level of communal activity that exceeded that of many of their hearing counterparts.

The breadth of activities found in *British Deaf News* shows that there were no physical reasons why deaf people should not be involved in virtually any leisure activity. When no evidence of particular activities can be found, this does not necessarily indicate an inability to participate; instead, it shows that deaf club members merely chose to take part in certain activities rather than others. This exercise of choice was influenced by factors such as local preferences and historical involvement in certain leisure pursuits, both amongst deaf people themselves and by the wider population. In their leisure lives, deaf people were as subject to the vagaries, fashions and trends of leisure as any other community or social group. Various activities that became popular in the wider world, such as the growth in overseas holidays from the 1960s onwards, were not closed to deaf people simply because of their deafness.

Conversely, there is nothing evident in the historical record that is overtly or uniquely 'deaf' in terms of what deaf people chose to do together, although some of the psychological and emotional benefits derived from these might have been greater. In general terms, the leisure activities of deaf people in north-west England do not seem markedly different from those one might expect to find being enjoyed by other social groups in the region during the post-war period or indeed by deaf people in other parts of the UK. Whilst the most popular activities such as organised trips and communal holidays might be enjoyed by other community groups, what appears distinctive about the involvement of deaf club members is the number and frequency of such events. The one aspect of leisure in which deaf people were somewhat more conservative in their choices was in their communal sporting activities. These were largely restricted to those one would expect to find in working-class communities, such as football, cricket, bowls and snooker. Even after a range of sports became more generally accessible from the 1970s onwards, deaf people did not appear to become involved in these as representatives of their deaf clubs as they had with other sports.

By joining a deaf club, members were able to pursue a range of leisure activities that suited their interests in the company of like-minded others, and which provided companionship and a variety of psychological benefits that were often absent from their daily lives. This absence was due in no small part to the communication difficulties that were an intrinsic part of deaf people's lives. However, although deaf people mostly engaged in the social aspects of leisure with other deaf people, deaf social life was not exclusively 'deaf only'. There are numerous examples of deaf people either actively engaging in social and sporting activities with hearing people, or choosing to attend the same events as audiences or observers. This indicates that a commonality of interests could be – and often was – shared by both deaf and hearing people. The

importance of these shared interests and activities is an important consideration when the issue of whether deafness should be seen as a disability is
discussed later.

Since the 1990s, the number of activities organised by deaf clubs has
decreased, as the deaf clubs themselves went into decline. Whether these
declines were symbiotic is not definitively proved by the data, but it seems
highly likely that the decline of both the clubs and their organised activities
were mutually motivated. In simple terms, deaf clubs lost their appeal for
certain elements of the deaf population. The reasons for this decline were
closely linked to the changing social habits of younger deaf people, as well as
changes in the way deaf children were educated. As the influx of new members
dried up, so the demographic profile of deaf clubs progressively became older,
membership numbers shrank and the historical record shows that as a consequence the number of activities organised by the clubs decreased. Deaf clubs
gradually came to be both the perceived and the actual refuge of older deaf
people, and participation in deaf club based sport in particular suffered as a
result. This decline was similar to that experienced by a variety of social clubs
across the north west, illustrating once again the way in which leisure trends in
the deaf community broadly mirrored those of the wider population.

Although this analysis has focused specifically on north-west England,
many of the conclusions drawn can be applied more broadly. Examples of
the specific leisure activities enjoyed by deaf people in the north west could
also be found being in other parts of the country. Where there were noticeable differences between the north west and other parts of Britain, these were
mostly in the sports that were pursued. For example, golf, squash and tennis
featured rarely in the reports from the north west but were to be found in the
sporting life of deaf people in other areas. On the other hand, some sports
rarely – if ever – featured in deaf sport anywhere in Britain; examples include
both codes of rugby, gymnastics and hockey. When the odd example was
found, these showed that these sports were more often pursued by individuals rather than as an organised or collective deaf club activity. This general
conformity of leisure helps to emphasise that a lack of hearing would not
necessarily produce a radically different world view in all aspects of life. The
picture produced by the evidence is of an active community whose members
regularly joined together to share their leisure time in a wide range of activities and interests. This communal activity continued until the last quarter of
the twentieth century, after which the traditional forms of deaf leisure activity declined (but did not disappear completely) in favour of more fragmented
socialising. In this, the deaf community showed itself to be no different than
other sections of society.

Attachment to the deaf club as a concept

Beyond the basic factual history of deaf leisure provided by *British Deaf News*, a number of qualitative issues arise which warrant closer discussion, as they help to emphasise the importance of leisure and sport in the wider social and cultural life of deaf people in Britain. The data drawn from *BDN* provides a unique insight into deaf life and gives rise to a reappraisal of certain aspects of the deaf community. First amongst these is a confirmation that the term 'deaf club' represents more than the physical premises within which the deaf club was housed. As Wise points out, 'home' is not necessarily just a place, but it is also possible to associate feelings of home with the presence of what he terms 'significant others'.[1] It was not until the late twentieth century that deaf clubs lost their position as the *de facto* homes of the deaf community; prior to losing this pre-eminence, deaf clubs constituted more than just a place where deaf people met. Bale's claim that attachment can not only be felt to a physical place but also to the concept of community engendered by that place can also be applied to deaf clubs.[2] Many of the activities took place away from the building in which the deaf club was based but these were just as much a part of 'going to the deaf club' as those events which were held within the club itself. So the idea of 'the deaf club' was as closely associated with the people and events that the term represented as it was to a geographical space. In reality, the deaf community has had no physical embodiment in the daily lives of adult deaf people, who largely spend their time apart from each other. As such, the deaf community represents a prime example of Anderson's concept of the 'imagined community'.[3]

Therefore, the existence of deaf clubs was vital to the development and maintenance of the notion of a deaf community, as they represented the main or indeed sole form of communion with others who shared similar experiences, outlooks and values. Where that communion was found was less important than having contact with the body of people who comprised the deaf club. For deaf club members, 'significant others' encompassed not only fellow members but also members of other deaf clubs, with whom they shared and expressed their communal culture and identity. For deaf people, the deaf clubs provided access to a community which extended well beyond the confines of the deaf club and which encompassed many more people than merely the local deaf population. In this way, the deaf community was promoted and maintained as a positive aspect of deaf people's lives, and through the community's shared activities deaf culture was preserved and passed on to new members.[4] Padden and others have claimed that it was only by conforming to the community's cultural norms that membership of the deaf community could be achieved.[5]

How these cultural identifiers were expressed within the context of shared leisure activities is quite clear. Put simply, deaf people chose to do certain things together; in doing so, these became part of their shared culture as deaf people. The sheer scale of communal deaf leisure uncovered here demonstrates the importance of leisure in the wider social and cultural life of deaf people not only in north-west England but across Britain.

Deaf clubs in decline

Somewhat perversely, the success of deaf clubs in bringing deaf people together may have been a primary contributor to their ultimate decline. That is because there is an important relationship to be seen between the degree of autonomy that the organisation of deaf clubs offered to deaf people and Bourdieu's concept of social and cultural capital.[6] Through the clubs' activities, the cultural elements of deaf social life were accessed and expressed, and these activities provided members with an important means by which to accrue social and cultural capital. Deaf clubs were the main means by which these types of capital were acquired by deaf people, as they were often the only places in which anything approaching a 'normal' social life could be found. By providing both social and cultural capital, the cultural aspects of deaf life eventually became more overtly important as the deaf community as a whole became more politicised. Deaf culture moved from being the way deaf people behaved naturally to something which was more explicitly treasured and celebrated.[7]

Evidence to support Bourdieu's argument that capital could also be accessed through activities that are specifically political can be found in the actions of deaf club members. The activities of deaf club members were largely self-determined, increasingly so during the post-war period. Deaf people ran the deaf clubs on a day-to-day basis and it was the members who largely determined the calendar of social events. Deaf clubs provided deaf people with opportunities to become politicised, through the exercise of choice in determining their communal social lives. Members formed and joined various committees, which were charged with taking responsibility for organising and financing a number of appropriate events and activities on behalf of the membership. For many deaf people, the exercise of such control over their own lives would have been a novel experience, having been subjected to an educational and welfare system which regarded them as needing care and which controlled and ordered many aspects of their daily lives. The clubs also played an important role in supporting the work of the deaf organisations, especially the British Deaf Association (BDA). Almost every club was effectively a local

BDA branch, providing officials for the organisation, and offering a route by which politically-active but geographically dispersed deaf people could join together. The actions of the BDA through their involvement in deaf clubs provided political capital for those members who took part in overtly political activities such as acting as Branch Secretary and voting in BDA elections. From the 1970s onwards, the growth in political activism amongst deaf people of all ages, but especially younger deaf people, gave rise to demands for equality in all aspects of their lives.[8] As Rose and Kiger state, 'when a minority group begins to re-evaluate its status, members also re-evaluate their notions of what the group deserves'.[9] Within the deaf community, one consequence of this re-evaluation was a broadening of both the scope and expectations of their leisure activities and forms of cultural expression.

Deaf clubs declined as a consequence of younger deaf people finding new forms of acquiring social capital that did not include membership of the local deaf club. The slow demise of the deaf clubs was not helped by changes in other aspects of deaf life that had the biggest impacts on younger deaf people, as they became more integrated into mainstream society. The natural progression route from the deaf schools into the clubs was lost as deaf children were increasingly taught alongside hearing pupils, rather than being educated discretely. The deaf schools themselves had served as a means of entry into the culture of deaf people and the larger deaf community. After schooldays were over, the deaf clubs allowed access to the community to be maintained, as well as providing an entry route for others. With educational integration came a greater exposure to mainstream culture, whilst an increased awareness of the options available for spending leisure time coincided with another of the entry routes into the deaf community disappearing. The replacement of the Missioner, based in the deaf clubs and an active propagandist for the benefits of membership amongst young deaf people, by a more detached Social Worker for Deaf People meant that this traditional means of access to both the deaf clubs and subsequently the deaf community was also lost. Emerging technology such as textphones, mobile phones and SMS, email and the internet all meant deaf people could keep in touch with each other instantly and on more than simply face-to-face terms. Subsequently the need to visit the deaf club in order to keep up to date with the latest news and gossip largely disappeared for younger deaf people. The combination of all three factors meant that the decline in deaf club membership was virtually inevitable unless some other means of advertising the clubs and drawing younger people into the clubs was introduced. The subsequent decline of the deaf clubs is evident in the diminishing levels of activity amongst virtually all deaf clubs across the UK, indicating alternative recruitment strategies were not introduced.

Puttnam's argument that the erosion of social networks results in a loss of shared social capital at least partially applied to deaf clubs, as they gradually became less influential as venues and providers of leisure opportunities, especially for younger deaf people.[10] However, the deaf community did not completely disintegrate in the ways Puttnam describes, but instead had become more fragmented by the end of the twentieth century. Although the deaf community sub-divided along the lines of class, age and political involvement, and deaf clubs became less important for some members, deaf people did not stop socialising with each other. Communal activity with other deaf people continued to be an important factor in community cohesion in a broader sense, but some of the activities changed (especially those of a non-sporting nature) and the primary venue of this social life moved away from its traditional home of the deaf club. By the mid-1990s, young deaf people were increasingly more likely to be found in pubs and nightclubs than their local deaf club. The clubs became instead the reserve of older deaf people, for whom mainstream leisure venues had never held the same attraction as the deaf club. Whilst it may be lamented by older deaf people, this change may not necessarily be of long-term damage to the deaf community. It is clear that whilst the deaf community changed in terms of how its members came together socially, it most emphatically did not disappear. In many ways, the deaf community in 1995 was stronger than at any period in its history, as members became more confident in being identified as deaf people and expressing their demands for their rights as human beings. Employment and education opportunities were enhanced by changes in government policy and there was a growing awareness amongst the hearing majority that many deaf people rejected the long held negative perceptions of deafness and its effects.

However, one unavoidable consequence of the changes in the deaf community and the decline of the deaf clubs was that some aspects of deaf culture came under threat. Deaf people from all sections of the community no longer joined together in the same numbers or as often. For example, the numerous trips previously made by deaf club members almost completely disappeared, and deaf clubs no longer hosted visits by other clubs as often as before. Although some of these traditional activities have been replaced by alternative forms of communal deaf leisure, there is often a distinct generation gap between those who take part and those who do not. For example, the annual Deaf Rally in Blackpool became increasingly an event that attracted only young deaf adults, rather than being the cross-community event it had been for most of the post-war period.[11] Indeed, the appeal of this particular event has been so great that it was rebranded as 'Deaf Rave' in the early twenty-first century. Many traditional forms of communal activity, such as the Wakes week holidays and Whit walks, have disappeared amongst the general population, and leisure patterns have changed dramatically since the 1970s. So the fact that changes occurred in the leisure activities of deaf people between 1945 and 1995 should not be surprising, nor that many traditional forms of entertainment were not as attractive to younger deaf people as they had been to previous generations. The changing nature of deaf leisure also shows once more that the deaf community responded to changing fashions in the majority hearing population and that deaf people's motivations for choosing certain leisure activities whilst rejecting others were no different from other social groups within society.

Deaf community or Deaf Nation? – the role of the deaf clubs

Several commentators have debated in recent years the possibility of the traditional deaf community evolving into a 'Deaf Nation' and the history of deaf people's leisure pursuits supports some of their arguments.[12] The Deaf Nation concept sees the deaf community at local, national and international levels developing into an effective global political structure, from its existing basis of a community of people linked by shared life experiences and outlooks. As a result of the increasing politicisation of the deaf community during the postwar period, it is claimed that the community is taking on the trappings of a nation and has begun to evolve beyond being merely a community. The analysis of deaf leisure activities provides evidence that at least some of the factors Anderson identified as being central to the nation-building process can be found within the deaf community. Anderson wrote '[the nation] is imagined as a community because… the nation is always conceived as a deep, horizontal comradeship'; the picture of the deaf community painted by the evidence of communal activity strongly suggests that 'the deaf community' could be substituted for 'the nation' in this quote and the sentiments would hold true.[13]

The philosophical concept of the deaf community has been as important to its members as its physical embodiment in the association known as 'the deaf club'. It is here that the argument that the deaf club constitutes 'home' and its members 'significant others' finds its most compelling evidence. Without the sense of identity and purpose that members of the deaf community have shared, the idea of a Deaf Nation could not have found support from the very heart of the community. Once the idea of a shared community was established, members of the community found a common identity. In some ways, it was almost inevitable that ideas of nationhood would eventually follow once the deaf community gained control over certain aspects of their lives and through this self-determination became more assertive in demanding their rights as equal members of society. It was through the political campaigning conducted by organisations such as the British Deaf Association and the National Union of the Deaf, through the pages of *British Deaf News* and in talks given in deaf clubs, that many deaf people first became politically active. The network of deaf clubs allowed these political campaigners to seek out and join with others with similar aims and to develop a national focus to their campaign. Anderson defines the nation as 'an imagined political community' that emerges from a number of smaller social groups or 'villages'.[14] Through their place at the forefront of the deaf community's political campaigning, deaf clubs might be seen as the 'villages' from which the 'imagined political community' that is at the heart of the Deaf Nation principle emerged.

Anderson contends that nationality arises when three cultural conceptions are no longer a central influence within a community: privileged access to the community by knowledge of language; the existence of a dominant external hierarchical system of control over society; a decline of the importance of religious faith in daily life.[15] All three factors have been important considerations throughout the history of the deaf community in Britain. The issue of language is the hardest to resolve in the context of the Deaf Nation, but some relevance can be seen. Deaf people had their preference for the visual/gestural mode of communication of sign language denied; developing speech and using hearing aids was imposed through the education they were subjected to and they had no legal recourse to services provided in sign language. Those who did not or could not learn to speak clearly and lip-read well were regarded as failures and incapable of fulfilling useful roles in society.[16] This argument was rejected in the deaf clubs. When deaf people were not subjected to outside pressures, their predominant and preferred form of communication was sign language and they enjoyed a full and rewarding social life as a result of having effective and meaningful communication with other people. It was only in the later years of the twentieth century that sign language began to be accepted by those outside the deaf community as a true language and the most appropriate means by which many deaf people could communicate with other people, whether deaf or hearing. The long process of accepting deaf people as full members of society, despite their not having full or effective use of the language of that society, had at least begun. Language also plays another important role in developing ideas of an alternative nationhood, as knowledge of a community's language is an essential pre-requisite for anyone wishing to gain membership of what Anderson terms 'pre-nation' communities.[17] Both the use of – and respect for – sign language have been equally essential for those hoping to enter the deaf community. So rather than being excluded from the nation of the hearing majority by their lack of English language skills, sign language users came to find themselves having the means by which they could develop their own ideas of nationhood, from which those who could not sign were excluded. Whether hearing people who can sign will have a role to play in the Deaf Nation will no doubt be as contentious an issue as it has been in discussions about deaf community membership.

The perceived control of deaf people's lives by hearing people has been the source of debate and argument throughout the deaf community's existence, and the demands for deaf self-determination and human rights grew as the deaf community became more politicised from the 1970s.[18] Much of this control was exercised through religious bodies, with church groups being the main providers of welfare and support for deaf people. Within the specific context of this research, the presence of an external hierarchy and the decline of religious influence in deaf life can both be seen. Anderson's 'dominant external hierarchy' was evident in the person of the Missioner who took control over many aspects of the lives of the deaf people in his care. The Missioners themselves were not rejected by the deaf community (and it must be acknowledged that many older deaf people remember their Missioners with some affection), but their influence did extend to virtually every aspect of a deaf person's life. As such, they acted as the representatives of what many saw as the hearing world's oppression of deaf people and it was this that was rejected. As Anderson notes, many nation states emerged from a sense of religious or colonial oppression and this has been a constant theme in deaf activism.[19] It was only after the transfer of deaf welfare to Social Services departments that the influence of religious groups began to dissipate to any degree and the change from Missioner to Social Worker for Deaf People also coincided with a growth in more widespread deaf political activism. The change did not come about as a direct result of pressure from deaf people, but it may have provided encouragement for those seeking to gain more control over their lives. The churches were not rejected outright, but much of what they had historically represented in terms of exerting control over the lives of deaf people was.

Another factor in the development of nationhood highlighted by Anderson is the role of newspapers as cultural product.[20] Despite the introduction of new technology which allows deaf people to communicate with each other more readily over distance, and the dissemination of information through television programmes aimed at deaf viewers, the deaf newspaper remained an important means of mass communication throughout much of the second half of the twentieth century. Members of the nation state do not have to meet in order to share a common bond of nationhood:

> [a nation] is *imagined* because the members of even the smallest nation will never know most of their fellow members, meet them or even hear of them, yet in the minds of each lives the image of their community.[21]

In this way, the image of the deaf community was both reflected and engendered through the pages of *British Deaf News*; after all, other than the temporary existence provided by attendance at a residential deaf school or a deaf club, the deaf community has no physical embodiment. It was through reading the gossip and news reported in *BDN* that many deaf people kept in touch with those community members they did not know, had not met nor even heard of. *BDN* allowed readers to keep in touch with deaf people with whom they had no other means of communication, and in doing so, the newspaper served as an important cultural tie within the community. As the nature and culture of the deaf community changed, this was mirrored in both the content and the purpose of *BDN*. For example, when the National Union of the Deaf began to campaign more directly for the rights of sign language users from the mid-1980s, the main deaf organisations followed suit and many deaf people became more politically astute and active as a result. This is reflected noticeably in the pages of *British Deaf News*, which became much more an organ of dissemination for the political activities of the British Deaf Association from 1980 onwards.

The notion of a single imagined deaf community has declined in recent years as community members have become more politicised, and this is reflected in the historical record of deaf leisure.[22] The Deaf Nation concept seems to be the logical consequence of the fragmenting of the deaf community illustrated by changes in members' leisure activities and this may well be the next stage in the development of what is presently regarded as 'the deaf community'. The imagined community of deaf people is well established and has developed in a number of new directions; it has rejected (but not yet overthrown) a dominant external hierarchy based in part on religious teachings; it has its own language in British Sign Language and its cultural products include *British Deaf News*. Although the continued existence of a community based on shared deafness is not disputed, this is no longer expressed in the same way through leisure activities that are shared by the whole community and centred in the deaf clubs. Through the informal gatherings at places they attended to receive welfare, deaf people built on the relationships and ideas of shared identity that had been formed at deaf schools. From these meetings, more structured social bodies emerged which eventually became the network of deaf clubs that are still in existence today. Without the deaf clubs in which to meet other deaf people and share leisure activities, the deaf community could not have developed and flourished. It was the success of deaf clubs in helping to maintain and enhance feelings of belonging to a community of deaf people that ultimately led to the diversification of that community, as younger deaf people become more empowered, confident and assertive.

The paradox of this situation is that the acceptance of the idea of the Deaf Nation grew during a period in which the traditional homes of the deaf community went into decline. Therefore, in many ways, deaf clubs were unwitting victims of their own success and their demise should be seen as an indication of progress amongst deaf people rather than signalling the end of the deaf community. Since the Second World War, the deaf community at grassroots level had changed from a community based primarily on shared social bonds to one that is just as closely aligned through overt political aspirations. As with many other groups within society, the social life of the deaf community is now more diverse than ever before. However, that communal social life has not disappeared; it has merely moved into other locations and involves alternative forms of social and cultural expression, in addition to the traditional homes and activities of the community. Although *BDN* no longer plays an important role in maintaining contact amongst younger deaf people, texts, MSN and email have become its natural successors and these play an even more important role in developing ideas of deaf identity through the independence they provide.

Deaf leisure and sport – challenging notions of disability

Most communities form on the basis of 'sameness' and one of the ways in which this sameness is celebrated is through shared leisure. Sport on the other hand celebrates sameness within a group but emphasises difference from outsiders, as represented by opponents. Analysing deaf leisure and sport therefore provides an opportunity to reassess who and what the 'deaf community' has been and how it has been constituted based on issues of sameness and difference evident in these activities. It is not intended to revisit here the theoretical models of community membership, but rather to use the history of deaf leisure to challenge the prevalent perception of deafness as a disability. The idea of deafness as a disability is one that has been rejected by the majority of the deaf community, and the evidence of deaf leisure and sport supports this rejection.[23] There is nothing in the available evidence to suggest that deaf people's social lives differed significantly from those of hearing people in terms of what they chose to do. In many respects, it was the way in which deaf club members collectively shared their leisure time, rather than what they chose to take part in, that marked them out as being different from other voluntary associations. Deaf clubs did not provide the escape *from* normality that is a motivating factor in all leisure activity; instead, the clubs provided an escape *into* a world of normality that could not be found in the outside world. In their everyday lives, deaf people were defined on the basis of their exclusion from the 'normal' world, and treated accordingly. They lived in a world in which their deafness marked them out as 'different'. Deaf people and hearing people could not generally communicate easily with each other and deaf people suffered as a consequence, not least in the way they were perceived. The majority of the hearing world saw deaf people as abnormal, deficient, handicapped or disabled and subjected to any number of similarly negative perceptions. Deaf people were deemed to be worthy of pity or charity, rather than being accepted and acknowledged as a distinct social and cultural group. Instead, the hearing majority's efforts were concentrated on finding ways to cure their deafness and thus remove the cause of their difference.

The alleviation of difference brought on by disability is at the centre of general attitudes towards people regarded as disabled. Oliver notes that 'disabled people continue to be portrayed as more or less than human, rarely as ordinary people doing ordinary things'.[24] In other words, disabled people are seen to be prevented from leading 'normal' or 'ordinary' lives by their disability. Oliver further argues that the notion of disability is then perpetuated by the imposition on and towards disabled people of an attitude of dependency.[25] The general perception that arises from this view is that if disabled people are to lead as 'normal' a life as possible, they cannot do so without the help of the 'able-bodied' majority. As the evidence from deaf leisure has shown, neither of these perceptions of disability can be applied to deaf people, particularly in the context of their social lives. They were not dependent on 'able-bodied' others (in the context of deafness, this would mean hearing people) for this social life, beyond using sign language interpreters for some events. Whilst certain aspects of the deaf clubs were initially managed by the Missioners and later the Social Workers for Deaf People, such as strategic financial matters, the organisation of the day-to-day running of the deaf clubs and the choice of club activities was placed in the hands of the members. Towards the end of the research period, all aspects of deaf club management were increasingly being made with the involvement of deaf people working alongside hearing specialists (such as accountants), rather than being the sole preserve of hearing people delegated to the task.[26]

As for being disabled through an inability to do ordinary things, the evidence of deaf people's leisure activity contradicts this entirely. The only difference in the way deaf people took part in certain leisure activities was the language of interaction. When some leisure activities overtly required sound or hearing, alternative forms of participation were found and numerous examples of such adaptations were found in *British Deaf News*. For example, before the days of subtitled popular films shown in mainstream cinemas, Liverpool Deaf Club showed foreign language films with English subtitles.[27] Plays were translated into sign language, and on occasion narrators were provided for those hearing people who were denied access by an inability to sign.[28] In addition to these examples, a wide range of other events were made accessible following the introduction of sign language interpreters during the later years of the research period.[29] Once events were made accessible, deaf people once again demonstrated their 'ordinariness' by attending those events that appealed to them, not just because they were accessible. Even before the availability of interpreters, deaf club members attended 'hearing' cultural events such as the theatre, cinema and even pop concerts.[30]

What is clear from the extensive evidence presented in *BDN* is that there is no foundation for claiming that deaf people were physically incapable of taking part in ordinary leisure activities. As has been demonstrated, these activities were equally attractive to both deaf and hearing people, and were often attended by both. As such, although individual events may have been seen as special occasions, they nevertheless constituted an ordinary way of filling available leisure time. The evidence clearly shows that whilst deaf people might not have taken part in every type of activity that hearing people did, those they did enjoy were no different to those of their hearing counterparts. The argument that deaf people should be regarded as disabled because of an inability to take part in ordinary events is refuted by the evidence of their engagement in leisure activities.

The analysis of deaf sport further contradicts the notion of deaf people being disabled. Aitchison contends that disabled people are excluded from mainstream leisure to some degree, and especially sport, and the majority of such provision is discrete rather than being integrated with non-disabled participants.[31] It is clear that this has not applied to deaf sportsmen and women, as they regularly and consistently took part in a variety of sports both alongside and in competition with 'able-bodied' (hearing) people. Deaf teams and individuals engaged in football, cricket, bowls, snooker and several other sports, as members of competitions and teams involving a majority of hearing players. In the case of football (the only sport in which deaf involvement has been extensively researched), some deaf players were of a sufficiently high standard to play professionally.[32] It must be accepted that deaf sportsmen and women have been regarded as disabled by hearing opponents and even teammates, but their ability to play alongside hearing players proves this perception to be wrong.[33] Deafness presents no physical barrier to taking part in any sport, as can be seen by the levels of involvement in the years since 1945. The only accommodation required as a result of participants being deaf is in the way a sport is controlled, with flags or lights being used instead of whistles or starting pistols for example.

Deaf involvement in sport has been essentially no different to that of hearing participants, although some deaf people regard certain team games to be of a higher standard when played by hearing people. It is claimed that because hearing competitors can call to each other without needing to look up, for instance to see where to place a pass or to identify opponents and teammates, that the game is quicker and therefore of a better quality. This has acted as an incentive for deaf sportsmen and women to choose to play alongside and against hearing people.[34] Although the range of sports deaf people took part in was limited to a degree, this appears largely to be due to issues of choice and access rather than because a lack of physical capability. For example, there was little evidence of deaf people in north-west England playing golf or squash. However, deaf people in other parts of the country did take up these sports, indicating that deafness in itself was no barrier. They were not excluded from mainstream sport; indeed, without involvement in hearing sport, the opportunities available to deaf sportsmen and women would not have had as extensive or rewarding. Nor were they solely dependent on hearing people for their sporting opportunities. Deaf people worked alongside hearing people in administering, organising and coaching various sports, and teams based in deaf clubs were run by the members. No matter which sports deaf people chose to take part in, the fact that they did so alongside hearing competitors, rather than being confined to competing with and against other deaf people, indicates that in sporting as well as leisure terms, deaf people should not be regarded as disabled.

Is deaf leisure different?

The final issue raised by this research questions whether the deaf community has shown any marked differences to other social or community groups in its use of leisure. Whether the answer is yes or no may depend on the role that leisure and sport are seen to play within society. Deaf people are distinct from other people simply because they are deaf, and so for this reason 'other social groups' can be taken to mean hearing people. Viewed as a means of filling free time, the deaf community has not used leisure or sport any differently to hearing people, in either the choice of activity or the reasons for those choices being made. It has been shown conclusively that deaf people took part in activities that were no different from those engaged in by hearing people. The motivational factors for choosing certain activities and sports were the same for both deaf and hearing: sociability, emotional rewards, and group and self-identity. If this were not the case, deaf people would not have taken part in as many communal events and activities as they did, nor in as much variety. The attraction of sport motivation identified by Holt in maintaining and strengthening existing social ties, as well as providing an opportunity for attracting others of a similar background into the social circle of the group or community, can equally be applied to the more general leisure pursuits of deaf people.[35]

Deaf people took part in leisure activities for the enjoyment these activities brought; the fact that they themselves were deaf was mostly incidental in terms of what they chose to do. The one exception was in their choice of companions and teammates. Deaf people chose to share so much of their leisure time in each other's company precisely because they were deaf. As happens in virtually every other leisure setting, people with shared goals and interests are drawn together to form social groups. In this respect, deaf people showed themselves to be no different to anyone else; they preferred the company of those with whom they shared interests and bonds. In doing so, the social ties between deaf people were maintained and extended, most notably in the number of trips made between deaf clubs. Where the deaf community's use of leisure might be considered to differ from that of other social groups was in the extent to which communal leisure was regarded as a means of cultural expression. However, although the activities themselves may have differed according to the particular community involved, the reasons why these groups gather together are the same. All groups who identify themselves as different or separate join with each other to express, maintain and pass on their cultural heritage, and this is not something that is unique to deaf people. The reasons why members of a community come together to celebrate those elements of their shared culture, history and heritage remain constant no matter what the basis of the community.

When leisure and sport are considered as more than merely ways of passing the time, then the answer to the question of whether deaf people used leisure and sport differently must be 'yes'. This is due to the singular position of the deaf clubs in deaf people's lives. Deaf clubs were not just a place for deaf people to meet up with each other; in many respects, the clubs acted as a surrogate home for their deaf members. These members in turn provided an extended surrogate family for each other – Wise's 'significant others'. The extensive leisure activities of the deaf clubs were as much a response to large numbers of deaf people coming together as they were a motivation for people to join the clubs. Deaf people (especially those who are sign language users) spend the vast majority of their lives isolated from those around them. A lack of effective communication, often even within their own families, meant they had few opportunities to engage in the type of everyday interaction and socialising the hearing world takes for granted. For other social groups, whether based in working men's clubs, political associations, sports clubs, or in community groups based on ethnic origin, their members had access to social lives away from or in addition to those found in their clubs. They could socialise informally with their families and relations, through work, or amongst friends and neighbours. Deaf people did not have access to the same network of readily available social intercourse that was a normal part of daily life for hearing people. It was only in the deaf clubs that any degree of normality could be found; communication was not a problem, they were not seen as disabled or in need of care as a result of being deaf, and they could share their time with people who had the same outlook and life experiences as themselves. The deaf clubs provided possibly the only place in a deaf person's life where he or she was not subjected to negative perceptions of deafness and deaf people. The attractiveness of the deaf clubs for deaf people can be seen from the number of events that were arranged through the clubs. If they had not been important to deaf people, the clubs would not have flourished as they so obviously did.

The clubs also provided opportunities for their members to enjoy activities they might not otherwise have had access to. For instance, travelling independently to various places and events was perfectly possible for deaf people to arrange for themselves and there is evidence of this happening throughout the research period. However, without the company of others with whom to share the experience, many of the social and emotional motivations and rewards of the event would be missing. The vast majority of reports found in *British Deaf News* suggest those taking such trips either enjoyed the company of fellow deaf travellers or that solo travellers had pre-arranged meetings with other deaf people whilst away. In providing deaf people with access to a rewarding social life, the deaf clubs were no different to any other social club. By offering their members a sanctuary from the hearing world in which they did not fit easily, deaf clubs provided a service that was markedly different from that of other social groups. Many deaf people simply did not have any other access to the type of social normality that the deaf clubs provided. The clubs did not offer an alternative form of socialisation; they provided the only rewarding form of socialisation for many deaf people.

What future for deaf clubs?

The ways in which deaf people previously engaged in shared leisure and sport is now largely consigned to history. Younger deaf people still socialise with each other and take part in shared leisure activities, but they do so in ways that are radically and fundamentally different from earlier deaf generations. However, whilst what they do might have changed, why and how they do it remains largely unaltered. Jeff Hill describes voluntary association as being at the very heart of leisure activity in Britain:

Of all the sectors in which British sports and leisure pursuits are to be found it is the voluntary – the one created by people themselves as part of everyday life – that is the most extensive and deeply embedded, reaching into the very fabric of social life.[36]

In the British deaf community, the main form of voluntary association from the mid-nineteenth century onwards was provided by the deaf clubs. However, both anecdotal evidence from deaf club members and the data acquired from the pages of *British Deaf News* indicate that deaf clubs have been in a state of decline for several years. Although it is not possible to give any definitive dates, trends indicate a steady reduction in activity and membership since around the mid-1980s. The deaf club is still an important factor in the maintenance of the deaf community, but mostly for older deaf people. Younger deaf people are now finding their own means of expressing their deaf identity and for them deaf culture no longer automatically involves being a member of the local deaf club.

The importance of the deaf clubs in the historical development of the deaf community cannot be overstated. Voluntary association was in many respects the rationale for the existence of deaf clubs; without the deaf clubs, it is hard to imagine where or how else deaf adults would have had the opportunity to come together in a mutually satisfying social environment. Without this contact, many deaf people would have had little or no fulfilling social life, or been able to derive the benefits that result from regular socialisation with others of a similar background, life experience and communication needs. It may well be true that the gradual decline of the deaf clubs indicates that they are no longer relevant to the lives of younger deaf people, but without the deaf clubs, it is hard to see how the deaf community could have existed in any meaningful form. Without deaf clubs, many deaf people would have had no contact with other deaf people, no access to sign language or the deaf community, and no means of accessing the culture and history of that community. As such, deaf clubs were a fundamental factor in the development and continued existence of the deaf community in Britain. Through their membership of deaf clubs, deaf people were able to fulfil the requirements of Hill's definition of leisure and 'reveal their authentic nature as autonomous human beings'.[37] In their shared leisure and sport activities, deaf people found a common purpose which then allowed them to become more empowered in other aspects of their lives. This study has also shown that when it came to enjoying themselves, deaf people were no different to any other section of society. In deciding which leisure activities they took part in and with whom, deaf club members found mutual satisfaction and a sense of community identity.

Deaf people in post-war Britain had no choice concerning the physical aspects of their deafness; they were audiologically deaf. However, they were able to exercise choice in dealing with the consequences of this deafness. The vast majority of deaf people have historically tried to combat their deafness by making use of hearing aids and other technological aids to be as 'hearing' as possible. Those deaf people who chose to accept and celebrate their deafness did so by associating with others of a similar background, usually through becoming members of deaf clubs. They did not gather together on the basis of shared disability; instead they chose to celebrate their deafness and their deaf culture as a positive and affirmative aspect of their lives. Consequently, membership of a deaf club facilitated developments beyond mere leisure, by providing access to increased self-identity and self worth, the opportunity for language acquisition and development, and routes into political activism. The consequence was access to a world in which social and cultural expression and fulfilment were available, and through which it was possible to gain a positive self-identity that counteracted the medical perspectives of deafness as a disability. The world of social activity provided by the deaf clubs enriched the lives of many deaf people and provided much more than just an escape from the pressures of daily life.

Notes

1   Wise, 'Home: territory and identity'
2   Bale, *Sport, space and the city*
3   Anderson, *Imagined communities*
4   Padden, 'The deaf community and the culture of deaf people'
5   Instances of the various models for determining membership of the deaf community were discussed in chapter two
6   Peillon, 'Bourdieu's field'
7   For example, see Brien, 'Is there a deaf culture?'; Erting and Johnson, *The Deaf Way*; Ladd, *Understanding deaf culture*
8   The early history of the resurgence in deaf political activism in Britain is given in Lee, *Deaf liberation*
9   Rose and Kiger, 'Intergroup relations', p. 524
10 Puttnam, *Bowling alone*
11 For insights into changes into the way the Deaf Rally was perceived by deaf people, compare *BDN*, 1965, pp. 65, 72, 75 with *BDN*, 1990, May, p. 20
12 Alker, 'The realities of nationhood'; Emery, 'The deaf nation, five years on'; P. Ladd, 'Emboldening the deaf nation'; Lawson 'Do we want one or multiple deaf nations?'; Turner, 'The deaf nation notion'
13 Anderson, *Imagined communities*, p. 16

14   *Ibid.*, p. 15
15   *Ibid.*, pp. 39–40
16   See Conrad, 'Towards a definition of oral success'
17   Anderson, *Imagined communities*, p. 20
18   Numerous examples are given throughout Lee, *Deaf liberation*
19   Anderson, *Imagined communities*, p. 19
20   *Ibid.*, pp. 39–40
21   *Ibid.*, p. 15
22   Alker, 'The realities of nationhood' , p. 79
23   Examples include Finkelstein, 'We are not disabled'; Lane, 'Do Deaf people have a disability?'; Corker, 'Deaf and disabled'
24   Oliver, *The politics of disablement*, p. 61
25   *Ibid.*, pp. 78–94
26   Hodson interview
27   *BDN*, 1960, pp. 89–90
28   An example of spoken narration being provided for a play performed in sign language was reported in *BDN*, 1960, p. 42
29   See for example *BDN*, 1970, p. 155, 220; 1980, p. 349; 1990, pp. 20, 21
30   *BDN*, 1965, p. 255
31   Aitchison, 'From leisure and disability to disability leisure'
32   Atherton *et al.*, *Deaf United*
33   Atherton, M., D. Russell and G.H. Turner, 'More than a match: the role of football in Britain's deaf community', *Soccer and Society* 2, 3 (2001), pp. 22–43
34   Examples of this attitude expressed by deaf footballers are given in Atherton *et al.*, *Deaf United*, pp. 68–70
35   Holt, *Sport and the British*, p. 347
36   Hill, *Sport, Leisure and culture*, p. 130
37   Hill, *Sport, Leisure and culture*, p. 130

Select Bibliography

Primary sources

Newspapers

British Deaf News 1955–1995
British Deaf Times 1945–1950

Secondary sources

Aitchison, C., 'From leisure and disability to disability leisure: developing data, definitions and discourses', *Disability and Society* 18, 7 (2003), pp. 955–969

Alker, D., 'The realities of nationhood', *Deaf Worlds* 18, 3 (2002), pp. 79–82

Ammons, D.K. and M.S. Miller, 'Sports, deafness and the family', in C.J. Erting and R. Johnson (eds), *The deaf way: perspectives from the International Conference on Deaf culture* (Washington DC: Gallaudet University Press, 1994), pp. 542–544

Anderson, B., *Imagined communities: reflections on the origin and spread of nationalism* (London: Verso, 1991)

Atherton, M., D. Russell and G.H. Turner, *Deaf United* (Coleford: Douglas McLean, 2000)

Baker-Shenk, C and C. Padden, *American Sign Language: a look at its history, structure and community* (Silver Springs, Maryland: TJ Publishers, 1978)

Bale, J., *Sport, space and the city* (London: Routledge, 1993)

Ballantyne, J. and J.A.M Martin, *Deafness* (Edinburgh: Livingstone, 1984)

Borsay, A., *Disability and Social Policy in Britain since 1750* (Basingstoke: Palgrave, 2005)

Bourke, J., *Working class cultures in Britain 1890–1960: gender, class, and ethnicity* (London: Routledge, 1993)

Brailsford, D., *Sport, time and society: the British at play* (London: Routledge, 1991)

Brennan, M., M. Colville and L. Lawson, *Words in hand: a structural analysis of the signs of British Sign Language* (Edinburgh: Moray House College of Education, 1980)

Brien, D., 'Is there a deaf culture?' in S. Gregory and G. Hartley (eds), *Constructing deafness* (Milton Keynes: Pinter Publishers, 1991), pp. 46–52

Campbell, J., 'Why papers of record are history', *British Journalism Review* 17, 59 (2006), pp. 59–64

Corker, M., *Deaf and disabled or deafness disabled?* (Buckingham: Open University Press, 1998)

Crosby, A., *History of Lancashire* (Darwen: Phillimore, 1998)

Crow, G. and G.A. Allan, *Community life* (Hemel Hempstead: Harvester Wheatsheaf, 1994)

Davis, L. J., *Enforcing normalcy: disability, deafness and the body* (London: Verso, 1995)

De Pauw, K.P. and S.J. Gavron, *Disability and sport* (Champaign Illinois: Human Kinetics, 1995)

Devas, M., 'Support and access in sports and leisure provision', *Disability and Society* 18, 2 (2003), pp. 231–245

Dhesi, A.S., 'Social capital and community development', *Community Development Journal* 35, 3 (2000), pp. 199–214

Dimmock, A., 'Sport and deaf people' in G. Taylor and J. Bishop (eds), *Being deaf: the experience of deafness* (London: Pinter Publishers, 1991), pp. 192–195

Dimmock, A., 'A brief history of the RAD', *Deaf History Journal Supplement X* (2001), pp. 16–24

Erting, C. J. and R. Johnson (eds), *The deaf way: perspectives from the international conference on deaf culture* (Washington DC: Gallaudet University Press, 1994)

Eyles, J., *Senses of place* (Warrington: Silverbrook, 1985)

Finkelstein, V., 'We are not disabled, you are' in S. Gregory and G.M. Hartley (eds), *Constructing deafness* (London: Pinter Publishers, 1991), pp. 265–271

B. Franklin and D. Murphy (eds), *Making the local news: local journalism in context* (London: Routledge, 1998)

Glover, M., 'Looking at the world through the eyes of…: reporting the "local" in daily, weekly and Sunday local newspapers' in B. Franklin and D. Murphy (eds), *Making the local news: local journalism in context* (London: Routledge, 1998), pp. 117–124

Grant, B., *The deaf advance* (Edinburgh: Pentland, 1990)

Gregory, S. and G.M. Hartley (eds), *Constructing deafness* (London: Pinter Publishers, 1991)

Harris, J., *The cultural meaning of deafness* (Aldershot: Avebury, 1995)

Higgins, P., *Outsiders in a hearing world* (London: Sage, 1980)

Hill, J., *Sport, leisure and culture in twentieth century Britain* (Basingstoke: Palgrave, 2002)

Hill, J. and J. Williams (eds), *Sport and identity in the north of England* (Keele: Keele University Press, 1996)

Holt, R., *Sport and the British: a modern history* (Oxford: Clarendon, 1989)

Hudson, J., *Wakes week* (Stroud: Alan Sutton, 1992)

Humphreys, R., *Sin, organized charity and the Poor Law in Victorian England* (Basingstoke: Macmillan, 1995)

Jackson, P., *Britain's deaf heritage* (Edinburgh: Pentland, 1990)

Jarvie, G. and J. Maguire, *Sport and leisure in social thought* (London: Routledge, 1994)

Knight, J., *Excluding attitudes: disabled people's experience of social exclusion* (London: Leonard Cheshire Foundation, 1999)

Kyle, J.G. and B. Woll, *Sign language: the study of deaf people and their language* (Cambridge: Cambridge University Press, 1985)

Ladd, P., *Understanding deaf culture: in search of deafhood* (London: Multicultural Matters, 2003)

Lane, H., R. Hofmeister and B. Bahan, *A journey into the DEAF-WORLD* (San Diego: DawnSignPress, 1996)

Lee, R. (ed.), *Deaf liberation* (London: National Union of the Deaf, 1992)

Lees, L. H., *The solidarity of strangers: the English Poor Law and the people, 1700–1948* (Cambridge: Cambridge University Press, 1998)

Loy, J.W. and G.S. Kenyon, *Sport, culture and society* (London: McMillan, 1969)

Lysons, K., 'The development of local voluntary societies for adult deaf persons in England' in S. Gregory and G.M. Hartley (eds), *Constructing deafness* (London: Pinter Publishers, 1991), pp. 235–238

McLoughlin, M.G., *A history of the education of the deaf in England* (Gosport: Ashford Colour Press, 1987)

Mitchell, D.T. and S. Snyder, *The body and physical difference: discourses of disability* (Ann Arbor: University of Michigan Press, 1997)

Oliver, M., *The politics of disablement* (London: Macmillan, 1990)

O'Neill, R., 'Manchester and Salford Adult Deaf and Dumb Benevolent Society', *Deaf History Journal* Supplement II (1997), pp. 15–31

Padden, C., 'The deaf community and deaf culture' in S. Gregory and G.M. Hartley (eds), *Constructing deafness* (London: Pinter Publishers, 1991), pp. 40–45

Padden, C. and H. Markowicz, 'Cultural conflicts between hearing and deaf communities' in A. Crammate and F. Crammate (eds), *Proceedings of the seventh World Congress of the World Federation of the Deaf* (Silver Springs, Maryland: National Association of the Deaf, 1976)

Parasnis, I. (ed.), *Cultural and language diversity and the deaf experience* (Cambridge: Cambridge University Press, 1996)

Polley, M., *Moving the goalposts: a history of sport and society since 1945* (London: Routledge, 1998)

Puttnam, R. D., *Bowling alone: the collapse and revival of American community* (New York: Simon and Schuster, 2000)

Rose, P. and G. Kiger, 'Intergroup relations: political action and identity in the deaf community', *Disability and Society* 10, 4 (1995), pp. 521–528

Russell, D., *Looking north; Northern England and the national imagination* (Manchester: Manchester University Press, 2004)

Sacks, O., *Seeing voices: a journey into the world of the deaf* (New York: Harper Collins, 1989)

Seguillon, D., 'The origins and consequences of the first World Games for the Deaf: Paris 1924', *The International Journal of the History of Sport* 19, 1 (2003), pp. 119–136

Shapely, P., *Charity and power in Victorian Manchester* (Manchester: The Cheetham Society, 2000)

Skelton, T. and G. Valentine, 'Political participation, political action and political identities: young D/deaf people's perspectives', *Space and Polity* 7, 2 (2003), pp. 117–134

Stewart, D., *Deaf sports: the impact of sports within the deaf community* (Washington DC: Gallaudet University Press, 1993)

Stokoe, W. C., 'Sign language structure: an outline of the visual communication system of the American deaf', *Studies in Linguistics Occasional Paper 8* (New York: Academic Press, 1960)

Stokoe, W. C. (ed.), *Sign and culture* (Silver Spring, Maryland: Linstok, 1980)

Stokoe, W.C., D.C. Casteline and C.G. Croneberg, *A dictionary of American Sign Language on linguistic principles* (Silver Spring, Maryland: Linstok Press, 1965)

Swain, J., S. French and C. Cameron, *Controversial issues in a disabling society* (Buckingham: Open University Press, 2003)

Taylor, G. and J. Bishop (eds), *Being deaf: the experience of deafness* (London: Pinter Publishers, 1991)

Tuan, Y-F., *Topophilia: a study of environmental perception, attitudes and values* (London: Prentice-Hall, 1974)

Van Cleve, J.V. (ed.), *Deaf history unveiled* (Washington, D.C.: Gallaudet University Press, 1993)

Walton, J.K., *Lancashire, a social history* (Manchester: Manchester University Press, 1987)

Walton, J.K., *Wonderland by the waves: a history of the seaside resorts of Lancashire* (Preston: Lancashire County Books, 1992)

Ward, A. and G. Tampubolon, 'Social capital, networks and leisure consumption', *The Sociological Review* 50, 2 (2002), pp. 155–180

Wise, J. M., 'Home: territory and identity', *Cultural Studies* 14, 2 (2000), pp. 295–310

Woll, B., J. Kyle and M. Deuchar (eds), *Perspectives on British Sign Language and deafness* (London: Croom Helm, 1981)

Wright, D., 'Learning disability and the New Poor Law in England, 1834–1867', *Disability and Society* 15, 5 (2000), pp. 731–745

Internet sources

www.bda.org.uk – The British Deaf Association

www.britishdeafsportscouncil.org.uk – British Deaf Sports Council

www.genuki.org.uk/big/eng/Paupers – The UK and Ireland Genealogical Information Service

www.royaldeaf.org.uk – Royal Association in Aid of Deaf People

Index

alcohol and drinking 44, 51, 62, 92, 110, 126, 139, 153

angling 97, 111, 150

athletics 96, 119–120, 143, 145, 148

badminton 142–143, 145, 149

billiards 142–143, 145, 149
  see also pool; snooker

bowls 95, 98, 115–116, 118–120, 143–147, 158, 170

British Deaf Amateur Sports Association 94–95
  see also British Deaf Sports Council

British Deaf Association 41–43, 47, 80, 132
  branches in deaf clubs 43, 138, 162
  foundation 42–43
  provider of communal holidays 132
  role in deaf sport 94

British Deaf News
  content 80–81, 172
  importance within deaf community 80–81, 83, 165
  origins of 77–81
  see also British Deaf Times

British Deaf Sports Council 94–96, 142, 147
  see also British Deaf Amateur Sports Association

British Deaf Times 75, 77, 80–82, 148
  see also British Deaf News

British Sign language
  interpreting 41–42, 47–48, 85, 91, 94, 135, 140–141, 146, 162, 169–170
  linguistic foundation 15–19, 129
  number of users 14
  official status within UK 17, 42

card games 90, 92, 96, 121, 125–126, 147

charity 44, 93, 138, 146, 169
  see also voluntary welfare; fundraising

chess 143–144, 148

cinema 134, 169
  deaf people visiting 7, 129, 170
  see also films

Comite International des Sports des Sourds 18

cricket 95, 115–116, 119–121, 142–143, 147–148, 152, 158, 170

cultural capital 66, 161–163

cultural product 25, 166–167

dances 90, 92, 96, 125–126, 135,

deaf choirs 93, 139

deaf clubs
  decline 10–11, 52, 66, 88, 105, 126, 139, 159, 161–163, 168, 174
  distribution across UK 88–90
  location in north-west England 107
  management 46, 83, 161, 169, 171
  membership 7, 9–11, 48–50, 54–55, 71, 89, 91, 105, 110, 126, 133, 135, 159, 174–175
  origins 33–34, 43–47
  as refuges from hearing world 50, 53, 153, 168
  role in development of deaf community 19–20, 48–51, 60, 63, 169
  social class 51–55
  as sources of social capital 65–66, 163
  as surrogate homes 53, 172

deaf community
  definitions and membership models 3–4, 7, 10, 13, 20–25, 28–29, 168
  differentiating from deaf non-sign language users 21–24

Lightning Source UK Ltd.
Milton Keynes UK
UKOW06f0954210216

268774UK00007B/107/P